YOU DON'T HAVE TO DIET!

Also by Dr Tom Sanders

The Vegetarian Healthy Diet Book
(*with Colin Spencer*)
The Food Revolution

Also by Peter Bazalgette

BBC Food Check
(*with David Edwards*)
The Food Revolution
The Big Food and Drink Book
(*with Michael Barry and Jilly Goolden*)

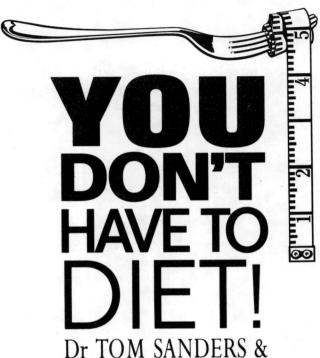

YOU DON'T HAVE TO DIET!

Dr TOM SANDERS &
PETER BAZALGETTE

BANTAM PRESS

LONDON · NEW YORK · TORONTO · SYDNEY · AUCKLAND

TRANSWORLD PUBLISHERS LTD
61–63 Uxbridge Road, London W5 5SA

TRANSWORLD PUBLISHERS (AUSTRALIA) PTY LTD
15–25 Helles Avenue, Moorebank, NSW 2170

TRANSWORLD PUBLISHERS (NZ) LTD
3 William Pickering Drive,
Albany, Auckland

Published 1994 by Bantam Press
a division of Transworld Publishers Ltd
Copyright © Peter Bazalgette and Dr Tom Sanders 1994

The right of Peter Bazalgette and Dr Tom Sanders to be identified
as authors of this work has been asserted in accordance
with sections 77 and 78 of the Copyright Designs and
Patents Act 1988.

A catalogue record for this book is available from the British
Library.

0593 021843

The cartoon on page 20 is reproduced with kind permission of *Private Eye*.
The food pyramid on page 66 is reproduced by kind permission of the
National Association of British and Irish Millers and the Dunn Nutrition
Laboratory.

This book is sold subject to the Standard Conditions of Sale
of Net Books and may not be re-sold in the UK below the net
price fixed by the publishers for the book.

All rights reserved. No part of this publication may
be reproduced, stored in a retrieval system, or
transmitted in any form or by any means,
electronic, mechanical, photocopying, recording
or otherwise, without the prior permission of
the publishers.

Typeset in Palatino and Gill Sans by
Chippendale Type Ltd, Otley, West Yorkshire
Printed in Great Britain by
Cox & Wyman Ltd, Reading, Berks.

CONTENTS

An exposé of the billion-pound diet industry, including
an analysis of best-selling diet books and an assessment
of diet foods and products.

Understanding our basic instincts about food and
pinpointing the influences that make us forget that
food should be about enjoyment and sustenance.
Plus fill in our questionnaire and discover how you
relate to your plate.

Plump people are actually healthier than skinny ones but
society now glorifies slimness. What are the real dangers
of being underweight or overweight?

Fat has become a dirty word, but in fact body fat is quite
natural and fat in our diet is essential. Fat is important
for maintaining good health. Too much fat is inadvisable,
but it can easily be corrected.

ACKNOWLEDGEMENTS

Dr Tom Sanders and Peter Bazalgette would like to thank the following for their help in the preparation of this book:

Dr A. Crisp
Broo Doherty
Hattie Ellis
Dr Elizabeth Evans
Tamara de Grassi
Tim Hincks
The Journal of Irreproducible Results
Dr H. Lacey
Mark Lucas
Cherie Martin
Ursula Mackenzie
Francesca Oakley
Bipin Patel
Lucie Pollard
Dr Sheela Reddy
Moyra Rose
Linda Sanders
Jane Thomas
Dr Janet Treasure
Lorna Todd
Lowri Turner
Jane Vigus
Mary Evans Young

CONVERSION TABLE

Weight	1 ounce	28.4 grams
	1 pound	453.6 grams
	1 stone	6.36 kilograms
	100 grams	3.53 ounces
	1 kilogram	2.2 pounds
Volume	1 pint	568 millilitres
	1 litre	1.76 pints
Height	1 inch	2.54 centimetres
	1 foot	30.5 centimetres
	1 centimetre	0.39 inches
	1 metre	3 feet 3 inches
Energy	1 kilocalorie (calorie)	4.19 kilojoules
	1 kilojoule	0.24 kilocalories

YOU DON'T HAVE TO DIET!

INTRODUCTION

Imagine for a moment that some scientist claimed that we breathe too much and that we should all hold our breath to lower our blood pressure. Imagine that this point of view was taken up enthusiastically by the newspapers, who encouraged us to breathe less and develop blue complexions. Suppose that blue complexions then became fashionable – fashion models almost stopped breathing altogether and the rest of us, women in particular, tried to do the same.

The trend would spread rapidly. Soon women would be attending 'BreathWatchers', and teenagers would be trying to suffocate themselves in their bedrooms. Other guilty people, despite their desperate desire to be blue, would indulge in breathing 'binges' and lose all grip of their self-control. Inevitably racketeers would move in with magical pills that would reduce our appetite for air, cans of 'lite' air for 'that blue look', exercises to take away our craving for oxygen and tight bands to wear round the chest to restrict the size of our inhalations.

Breath Control would soon grow into a billion-dollar industry. Women who had achieved really blue complexions would boast, 'I feel like a new person,' and gain in self-confidence as they were showered with compliments. No longer would they be ashamed of an ugly pink complexion. Men would then find them attractive because they'd resemble the sensuous blue-skinned models appearing in girlie and fashion magazines.

All a joke? Yes, but a serious joke. It was written recently by an American witnessing what the diet industry is doing to people in the Western world. Once you replace breathing with eating you have a perfect description of our society in the 1990s. We have reached a stage at which a perfectly normal function – a highly pleasurable one, too – gives rise to mass neurosis. Eating is something to feel guilty about and it has become almost normal to be 'on a diet'. Many of us now binge and diet in succession, and a number of diseases are being caused by this unnatural behaviour. But we are the victims of a huge confidence trick. The truth is that you don't have to diet. Let's begin by exposing those who tell us that we do.

1 THE DIET RACKET

The diet industry is damaging both our health and our wealth as we waste larger and larger sums of money on products which do us no good. It particularly exploits women by encouraging the pursuit of unhealthy slenderness.

When we go on a diet we are more than likely to be fed a succession of half-truths and bogus science. Here are the top ten myths:

1. All dietary fat is bad.
2. Plumpness is unhealthy.
3. Skinniness is healthy.
4. Fat can be lost rapidly and safely.
5. There is a special, female fat called 'cellulite'.
6. Cellulite fat is caused by toxins.
7. You can spot-reduce fat, particularly on the hips and thighs.
8. Particular foods or combinations of foods can boost metabolism and speed up weight-loss.
9. Women under 50 are at real risk from heart disease.
10. Dieting is a healthy activity.

Walk into any bookshop, pick up almost any diet book (there will be no shortage of choice) and sample the opening chapter. The chances are that at least three of these myths will be woven into it. No diet book has ever sold well without a gimmick. No gimmick, by definition, has any real value and many are outright frauds – bogus science, miracle cures and magic substances (invariably from a South American tribe).

Our appetite for these sorts of fantasies seems to be limitless. Their perpetrators enrich themselves at our expense, exploiting our obsessions with weight, shape and appearance. Britain's slimming industry – misleading books, expensive and sometimes fraudulent products and dubious clinics – is now taking more than a billion pounds off us a year. Not only is the money wasted; the products and advice can be harmful.

What is the matter with us? Why are we taken in by shysters no different from the pedlars of the Wild West with their snake oil? Why do we allow the diet industry to cash in by selling us powders and snack bars at inflated prices? Later we examine why so many of us get fat and how our attitude to food is ever more neurotic. But, first, in this chapter, we are going to expose the self-appointed gurus of the diet trade. Cigarette companies, toy manufacturers, fashion designers, diet book authors, pill-pushers, high street chemists, slimming 'clinics' and plain crooks – they all play their part in this miserable business. Why have we developed a fear of food? What are the influences in society that cause millions of perfectly healthy teenagers – particularly girls – to decide that they need to 'go on a diet'? How did the cult of thinness start?

Smoke Gets in Her Eyes

Perhaps the most surreptitious 'thin' influence comes from the tobacco industry. Historically smoking was presented as a masculine activity, and cigarette manufacturers had difficulty selling their products to women. But in the 1920s the American brand Lucky Strike came up with the slogan 'Reach for a Lucky, not for a sweet'. For the first time cigarettes were being aimed at women and associated with slimness. Cigarettes came to be perceived as the key to a man's world. For women to succeed they had to cast off feminine looks, to dress and behave like men. They soon became associated with the slim-suited glamour of the likes of Bette Davis, Lana Turner and Greta Garbo. All were frequently seen smoking elegantly in films. In *To Have and Have Not* Lauren Bacall actually played a character called 'Slim' and uttered the immortal line, 'Just put your lips together and blow'.

It is true that smokers tend to be slimmer. Smoking can reduce appetite and sully the taste buds by dulling pleasurable food flavours. Nicotine is also a stimulant that can help burn calories. But smokers are also more likely to die of lung cancer and heart disease. Plump people aren't. In fact, on average, cigarette smokers live fifteen years fewer than nonsmokers.

The tobacco industry was not slow to capitalize on our desire to be thin. Brands were launched in Britain with names such as Silva Thins and Slim Kings. Virginia Slims were advertised in the United States with the strapline, 'Slimmer than the fat cigarettes that men smoke'. Cigarettes aimed at women are still longer and lighter, and – where advertising is still allowed – tall thin models are seen smoking them. Perhaps the ultimate contradiction in terms was when cigarette manufacturers started sponsoring tennis tournaments and got the colours of their packaging onto the clothes of top players such as Martina Navratilova. Here cigarettes could be linked to female slimness, fitness and health all in one go. In Britain cigarette advertising is now banned from magazines which have a quarter or more of their readership under the age of 25. But the influence remains. It is clear that the tobacco industry still targets women with a particular, slim style of cigarette. And whereas smoking has declined rapidly as a habit amongst men it has recently shown an increase amongst women. At the same time lung cancer has risen amongst women and fallen amongst men. Does thin still equal healthy? Did it ever? The pursuit of slenderness via smoking has taken a terrible toll. But it is not the only fashion to have glorified thinness.

Dead Fashionable

Rubens painted plump curvaceous women, considered in their time to be very sexy. The Victorians were also proud to be plump, favouring women of a similar shape and accentuating natural female traits such as large hips. But in the twentieth century, certainly since the 1920s, thin has been in. It would be futile to enter into a chicken-and-egg debate about whether the fashion industry originally created this trend or merely followed it. What is undeniably true is that fashion designers on both sides of the Atlantic since the 1960s have created the cult of the super-thin model.

Researchers at the American University in Washington, DC, have recently followed up a survey of Miss America contestants and *Playboy* centrefold models. The original study, between 1959 and 1978, showed a consistent year-by-year decrease in body size and weight. The latest study shows that since then Miss America contestants have continued to reduce in weight while the *Playboy* models have remained very thin, levelling off at between 13 per cent and 19 per cent below the expected weight for someone of their height and age. The researchers concluded that the levelling off is because the models cannot get any lighter without dying. And they point out that being 15 per cent below your expected body weight is a major criterion for anorexia nervosa. So there is nothing healthy about these 'ideal' women.

Whether in soft-porn magazines, fashion features or advertisements, adult women and teenage girls are bombarded with a bizarre image of the female form. This androgynous creature often has no hips or breasts to speak of, and so hardly any natural, feminine characteristics.

Kellogg's Special K television advertisements have used a model so slim as to be entirely unrealistic for the vast majority of those who buy the cereal. There are low-fat spreads, such as St Ivel Gold, which adopt the same technique, as do other foods aimed at slimmers, such as Ryvita. Many foodstuffs are now advertised as though slimness rather than sustenance or (horror of horrors) enjoyment is all that eating is about.

In 1993 *Vogue* was attacked for publishing pornography when the waif-like model Kate Moss posed in lingerie. It gave rise to a telling parody in *Private Eye* (Figure 1.1, overleaf).

From Twiggy in the 1960s to Kate Moss in the 1990s the boyish, breastless and small-bottomed top models seem anything but feminine. To help achieve this, girls of 14 or 15 years of age have sometimes been used on shoots. And thus it has become desirable – and literally fashionable – to be thin. Most models are size 10–12. The average size for British women is 16. Why should some parts of the fashion industry want, in effect, to de-sex women? Some observers of the fashion industry point to the influence of gay designers whose clothes and models reflect what they find attractive. They have encouraged, if not created, a new aesthetic for women: the slim androgyne. But the aesthetics of all designers apparently dictate that clothes look better on a tall thin body. Fashion, says the fashion writer Lowri Turner, is about ideals. Beauty is about exclusivity. So models cannot look like the majority.

The way the fashion industry operates also promulgates an unrealistic super-thin feminine ideal. Fashion photography for magazines is usually carried out months before the clothes actually reach the high street. So 'samples' are specially run up. These are always made in a small size, 10 or 12. Even when newspapers publish fashion features about clothes already available they invariably pick sizes 10

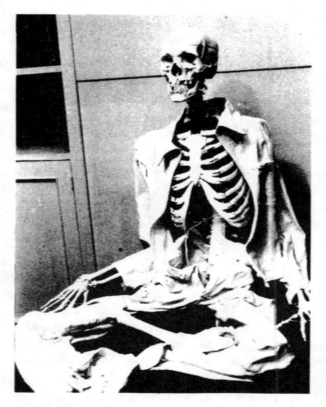

Figure 1.1

or 12 as the examples. Indeed, larger clothes (inaccurately called 'outsize' when they are only size 16) are often badly made because larger women can suffer from such low self-esteem, that they spend little on and expect little from such clothes.

Nowadays fashion photographs themselves can be touched up afterwards to remove stomach creases and any sign of normal flesh. Models are carefully posed as well. Fuller-bodied women are told to breathe in and are photographed sitting down. Breasts are pulled up by running Sellotape under them and under the arms.

Hence the absurdly unrealistic female icon that has emerged. What is the reality behind it? Just as some *Playboy* models and Miss America contestants are almost certainly anorectic, so many British models are themselves the victims of this bizarre trade in fantasy. When busts came into fashion (briefly) in the late 1980s quite a few catwalk models had breast implants. Many lost sensitivity in their breasts and didn't realize if their blouses had come undone mid-show. They would continue, unaware, down the catwalk. To add injury to insult, there is now a cancer scare about the safety of such implants. Eating disorders amongst models are widespread (estimates by insiders range from 20 per cent to 50 per cent). It is not unusual for a group of models to disappear to the toilet after a meal ostensibly to powder their noses. What they actually do *en masse* is make themselves throw up. The 'super-model' of the 1980s, Margaux Hemingway, has now come clean and admitted in public that she did the same. In pursuit of the 'perfect' figure she became bulimic. We are all aware of how painfully thin Princess Diana was at one time. It has been reported that she also was bulimic. Lest anyone should doubt how unhealthy thin can be, compare the glowing animated Diana of normal weight on coffee-mugs commemorating the royal wedding in 1981 with the gaunt sombre-looking figure we became more familiar with a few years later.

The fashion industry is responsible for perpetrating a perverted view of the ideal woman. This appalling distortion has a huge influence, not least by way of the slender clothes that women feel obliged to try to get into. In 1992, a 15-year-old girl committed suicide, having said that one cause of her unhappiness was being bullied at school for being size 14. Perhaps most worrying of all, eating disorders are no longer merely a teenage phenomenon. Eating disorder clinics admit girls as young as 9 who have been persuaded that they are overweight, while overall 60 per cent of us think we are overweight. The reality is that only 40 per cent of us are (from even the most stringent health point of view). But the malign influence of the fashion industry is by no means the only one.

Dolly Mixtures

When we saw an exercise video in the high-street stores – *Dance! Workout with Barbie* – it set us thinking. On the cover it shows the familiar, stick-insect figure of Barbie doing a dance exercise. In the video it claims the exercise programmes are for children over 5. Exercise videos are rather like diet books, presented by slim women with an air of fanaticism, all done in the name of the perfect figure. But what effect can such activities have on pre-pubescent girls? What sort of a role model do fashion dolls represent?

We have analysed three of the most popular dolls given to young girls at the moment. There is hardly a family in Britain that has not bought either a Sindy, a Barbie or a Little Mermaid. We first measured their height, hips, waist and bust (Table 1.1).

	Barbie	Sindy	Little Mermaid
	(cm)	(cm)	(cm)
Height	28	28	23.5
Hips	12	12	8
Waist	7	7	6.8
Bust	12	12.5	10.5

Table 1.1

We then took these measurements and worked out what sort of body they would represent for a woman of average height – 5 feet 4 inches (Table 1.2). The first column below shows what the vital statistics are for a normal healthy woman of this height.

	Normal 5'4" woman	Barbie	Sindy	Little Mermaid
	(inches)	(inches)	(inches)	(inches)
Hips	38	27.5	27.5	21.7
Waist	26	16	16	18.5
Bust	34/36	27	28.5	28.5
Inside leg	28/30	32	32	(Bent leg – not measured)

Table 1.2

These statistics, not vital in any sense, reveal that the toy industry is doing just the same as the fashion industry: presenting a bizarre and distorted feminine ideal. Though at least the toy manufacturers are doing it to plastic dolls rather than to real people. The dolls all have tiny hips by comparison with real women, tiny waists, much smaller busts and exaggerated inside leg measurements. We can only guess the effect this propaganda has on small girls. But it puts the emergence of 9-year-old anorectics into perspective. With pressure to be thin all around our children it means that parents should now be extremely careful what they say in the home. How many mothers have audible conversations about what sort of figure their young daughters are going to have. Will her thighs slim down? Will her bum be too big? Such apparently innocent remarks, on top of everything else, could end up being dangerous.

Indeed, the following statistics tell an alarming story. A 1983 survey published by the Department of Health found that about 5 per cent of 14-year-old girls were trying to lose weight. A similar figure of 6 per cent for 15–18-year-old girls was reported as long ago as 1985. Disturbing recent research by Jane Thomas at King's College, London, reveals that among 12 and 13-year-olds 22 per cent of boys and 39 per cent of girls want to lose weight and that 8 per cent and 16 per cent respectively were currently changing their diet to lose weight. As obesity is rare among this age group, most of these children don't need to lose weight. This trend was confirmed when Salwa El-Jabche at King's College investigated children who had been attending slimming clubs. Obesity is normally defined as being more than 20 per cent of the standard weight for height – it is a technical measurement of those who are overweight. She found that 32 per cent of girls aged 12-16 years attending slimming clubs were not obese and some of the children who were going to slimming clubs were not overweight at all. **Children and young people of this age do not belong in slimming clubs anyway.**

Obesity is not only rare among children; few teenagers experience it either. Table 1.3 (from a government survey carried out in 1991) shows that obesity is more prevalent with increasing age.

Age	16–24	25–34	35–44	45–54	55–64	65–74
% who are obese						
MEN	5	8	15	17	19	14
WOMEN	6	12	12	22	25	19

Source: OPCS 1993
Table 1.3

Why is the vogue for slimming increasing among school-children? We have looked at the pressure from the fashion industry and the strange stereotypes sold by the toy manufacturers. Dr Rose Dawson, who runs a centre for children with eating disorders, says that many of the children she sees also have mothers who are fanatical about diet and fitness.

Hundreds of thousands of young people are now dieting who do not need to. The prevalence of eating disorders and people who are seriously underweight has now emerged as a major health problem. Around 15 per cent of young women are now underweight. In schools, as elsewhere, the diet obsession has now taken hold.

Proud to Be Plump

Health obsessions are also responsible for the pursuit of slenderness. It is certainly unhealthy to be very fat, but the health hazards of being pleasantly plump are slight. In fact, for women there are actually health advantages in being plump (see Chapter 3).

We are constantly bombarded with information telling us the dangers of being fat, particularly with regard to heart disease. It is true that heart disease is a major cause of ill health among men, but it is not among women. And women are fatter by nature. Even with men most experts do not regard obesity specifically as a risk factor for heart disease. Only if a person has some other abnormality such as diabetes or high blood pressure does controlling body weight become important.

We are told that the extra body weight caused by the accumulation of fat puts a strain on the heart. While severe obesity certainly puts a strain on virtually everything in the body, moderate obesity does not. In fact, when people are merely plump, their hearts have to work harder when they are taking exercise. This is thought to be good for the heart. It probably explains why fat people are more likely to survive a heart attack than thin people. (For more information on plumpness and obesity, see Chapter 3.)

Fatness in women confers a number of benefits to health. Fat women are less likely to suffer from early menopause, heart disease and osteoporosis than thin women. On the other hand, women who become anorectic suffer from high blood-cholesterol levels that increase their risk of heart disease.

It is true that, as a nation, we are getting steadily heavier. At the extreme end of the scale this is a cause for concern. But it is crucial to understand that plumpness is healthier than skinniness. This is what the medical evidence shows. But it is the opposite of what we are normally told. A professor of nutrition, Donald Naismith, believes that simplistic health messages carry dangers. So that what is regarded as good advice for middle-aged men (lose weight, slim down) may not be such good advice for women or the young. Particularly when taken up with the vengeance some women and young people now apply to their diets.

Diet Books – Magic and Myths

If you have ever looked on the shelf of bestsellers in a high-street bookshop or cast your eye over the top-selling books listed in the newspapers, you will know how popular diet books are. The successful recipe for a diet book is:

- a gimmick or 'magic' formula
- the promise of rapid weight-loss or change of body shape
- a slim role-model authoress

It has been estimated that as many as one in five women, at any given time, are 'on a diet'. Many of them will be following the regime in a diet book. And yet, at the same time, Britain is increasingly becoming a nation of fatties. In 1980, 1987 and 1991 the Government surveyed our weight in Britain (Table 1.4). The survey discovered that obesity is growing.

	Obesity Survey	
1980	8% of women	6% of men
1987	12% of women	8% of men
1991	16% of women	13% of men

Table 1.4

While sales of diet books and magazines are spiralling upwards, so, too, is the weight of the nation. What does this say for the efficacy of the diets? In 1990 *Slimmer* magazine was also surveying weights – in this case, those of its readership. Their average weight was 11 stone 5 pounds, and their average height was 5 feet 4½ inches They were certainly plump, but how many needed to lose weight for their health's sake? We will sort out the confusion about what is a healthy weight in Chapter 3. But it is extremely difficult to get an honest answer to this question from diet books.

Most diet books work in the sense that they usually offer a short-term programme of restricted calorie-intake that can lead to weight-loss. They usually claim rapid weight-loss because we all enjoy seeing results and feeling that we're achieving something. But rapid weight-loss can be harmful:

- it can seriously weaken bones through loss of minerals
- it increases the risks of gout, gallstones and heart disease
- it damages the normal mechanisms that help control our body weight so that weight is regained more easily afterwards

Gradual weight-loss, coupled with learning how to moderate our food intake and activity level *for good*, is the only way to avoid the damaging cycle of weight-gain and weight-loss that many people suffer from (known as yo-yo-ng or weight cycling). Losing weight in the short term is rather easier than keeping it off in the long run. This is where the majority of diet books fail completely. They offer a short-term regime but do nothing to help us permanently. On the contrary, they offer false hope, encourage faddy eating and ensnare women in the diet trap. We have analysed some of the recent bestsellers to see how valid they are.

Rosemary Conley's Hip and Thigh Diet

Rosemary Conley's Hip and Thigh Diet has sold more than 2 million copies since its publication in 1988. It has been a publishing phenomenon. The second edition, *Rosemary*

Conley's Complete Hip and Thigh Diet, contains many letters from highly satisfied dieters who write to thank the author and praise her book. The book combines a low-fat diet with exercises. These are the reservations we have about the *Hip and Thigh Diet*:

1. There is the strong implication that this low-fat diet enables you to spot-reduce fat from your hips and thighs (**'we really can spot reduce our bodies, and not just on hips and thighs'**). And there are statistics claiming that dieters (who measured themselves) lose proportionately more earlier from these areas of the body. In fact, when dieting, our bodies lose fat from inside the abdominal cavity first, then from the face and between the shoulderblades, and then from the hips and thighs. At King's College, London, we carried out a comparison between a standard weight-reducing diet of 1000 to 1200 calories and the figures published in the *Hip and Thigh Diet*. It showed that the pattern of weight-loss was the same for both diets and that the most inches were actually lost from the waist rather than the hips and thighs. And as many inches were lost from the bust as from the hips.

   'I knew I'd lost weight . . . But it was unbelievable how the *inches* had disappeared, particularly from my hips and thighs . . . I couldn't believe what I was seeing.'

   This is how the author describes the first time she went on her low-fat diet. But we're sorry, Rosemary, there is no magic formula, nor has it anything to do with the nature of the diet. If we consume fewer calories, we lose weight. There is no good scientific evidence to show that low-fat diets do not lead to particular weight-loss from the hips and the thighs.

2. 'Never have I lost so much so easily and quickly!' 'I have never had so much success so quickly as on this diet.' 'It's great! This diet really does work!'

No doubt Rosemary Conley's many satisfied dieters quoted in her book did lose weight while following the low-fat diet, although none of the endorsements is medically verified, nor is it said what happened to the correspondents in the long term. But a scientifically validated study in Canada (by Norman Boyd at Ludwig Institute for Cancer Research in Toronto) showed that the majority of women on low-fat diets do not achieve long-term weight-reduction. Moreover, Professor Walter Willett at the Harvard School of Public Health says that controlled trials have failed to show that low-fat diets lead to long-term weight-loss. You can put on weight eating an excess of carbohydrate as well as an excess of fat. So, although we should not eat too many saturated fats for our health's sake, there is no magic in cutting fats right out.

3. This book gives little or no advice as to which of us actually need to lose weight for health reasons and which of us do not. It is characteristic of people with eating disorders to think they need to lose weight when in fact they are dangerously underweight. All diet books should help us check whether we are already a healthy weight and do not need to diet. If we still wish to diet for reasons of fashion and appearance, then they should warn us what the safe limits are for weight-reduction. This is not difficult to work out (see Chapter 3). It is interesting to note that Rosemary Conley was a healthy weight *before* she first embarked on her low-fat diet.

4. 'In more technical terms cellulite is a modified form of fat tissue to be found just below the surface of the skin.'

The *Hip and Thigh Diet* perpetuates the idea that there is a particular kind of female fat called cellulite. However, this term has no medical status whatsoever. The term was invented by French cosmetics manufacturers to help them sell more cream products for 'cellulite removal'. The plain fact is that women's thighs are prone to fat deposits just below the skin. It is entirely natural. The fat can become dimpled in appearance, which many women dislike. But it is not a **'storehouse for waste products'**, as Rosemary Conley claims, nor is it an ideal location for **'toxic waste products'** (see p.115 for an explanation of why thigh fat is dimpled). Junk food, apparently, **'encourages the deposit of fat'**. But what is junk food? And to continue, as Rosemary Conley does, that **'foods such as sugar, salt, spices, fat and alcohol can therefore aggravate a cellulite condition by cluttering up the system with additional waste matter'** is absolute rubbish. (Though we note that two alcoholic drinks per day are allowed on the diet.)

5. **'I could actually feel the nodules of fat cells disintegrating after a few weeks of applying cream daily, and the improvement became more and more obvious as I continued.'**

Having bought the cosmetics industry's fallacy that cellulite is a special type of fat, Rosemary Conley is then persuaded to apply one of their creams to her thighs. There might be an extremely marginal benefit from slightly increased blood-flow after application of such a cream. But it is wrong to suggest that fat cells **'disintegrate'** when cream is rubbed in. We believe such creams are a waste of money.

6. The book is mistaken about how much fat we should eat every day:

'The average consumption of fat in the Western world

at the present time is 130 grams (over 4½ ounces) a day per person.'

It goes on to suggest that we only need 5 grams of fat a day. In fact the average intake of fat is 90 grams for men and 80 grams for women, as the Department of Health's 1991 *Diet and Nutritional Survey of British Adults* makes clear. Experts on fat agree, and the World Health Organization has now stated that we need about 30 grams a day in order to be sure of getting the fats we need, and the vitamins, too. Some vitamins are best absorbed by our bodies when actually eaten with fats. We need to consume at least 5 grams of *essential fatty acids* such as polyunsaturates every day because our bodies cannot manufacture them. Rosemary Conley appears to have confused this figure with *total* fats. She does then make it clear that her diet does not, in fact, offer as little as 5 grams of fat a day. A good thing, too. And, by the way, butter is typically 81 per cent fat, not 99 per cent as the *Hip and Thigh Diet* says.

7. **'A man in his late forties is five times more likely to die of heart disease than a woman of the same age. But it would be a mistake for women to regard themselves as reasonably "safe", because after the menopause a woman loses the protective effect of her hormones and her chances of suffering from heart disease are almost equal to a man's.'**

It is true that a man in his late forties is much more likely to die of heart disease than a woman of the same age. It is also true that this changes after the menopause when a woman loses the protective effect of her hormones. But this is less to do with fatness and more connected to hormonal changes. These can lead to a rise in blood-cholesterol levels, however fat or thin you are.

'In recent years there has in fact been an increased

incidence of heart disease in women in their thirties and forties.'

This is not correct. Heart disease is very rare in women under the age of 50. What is more, rates of heart disease amongst women have been falling despite the rise in obesity. Younger women most at risk are those who have a combination of three factors: they smoke, they take the Pill and they have high blood pressure. A few severely obese women may run the risk of heart disease, but this is more to do with the association of obesity with diabetes and high blood pressure than with fatness itself.

8. **'I have given you a list of strictly forbidden foods within this chapter to enable you to make a definite resolution, before you begin the diet, to ban them totally from your life!'**

Among the items on the **'forbidden list'** are all yellow spreads and fatty fish. The oil in fatty fish may actually help prevent heart disease. Not only are these fats and oils in moderation a valuable part of any diet, but the **'forbidden list'** implies that there are **'good'** and **'bad'** foods. This is contrary to current thinking about nutrition which encourages a balanced range of foods rather than faddy obsessions with particular foods. The British Heart Foundation does not recommend the diet itself for those who want to learn how to eat healthily.

Why egg yolks are also forbidden we are not sure. They may contain 10 grams of fat each but they are high in protein and vitamins. To suggest that you should never eat fatty fish or egg yolks is bad dietary advice (we note that fatty fish was dropped from the **'forbidden list'** in the *Complete Hip and Thigh Diet*). To suggest as the author does that you should never eat cheese (except low-fat cottage cheese) is an appalling sentence that takes much of the pleasure out of eating. Cheese is delicious.

Overall Verdict: *Rosemary Conley's Hip and Thigh Diet* does not assess whether its individual readers need to lose weight. It perpetuates the myth that cellulite is caused by toxic substances. It implies that you can spot-reduce fat from the hips and thighs. It encourages faddy eating and exaggerates the health risk of fatness in women.

The Hay Diet

Dr William Hay invented 'food combining' in the early years of this century, long before modern medicine and nutrition and the detailed knowledge we now have about how our bodies work. He believed that disease resulted from the accumulation of toxins and acid waste in our bodies. He himself suffered from a kidney complaint – Bright's disease – which he thought could be cured by diet. (In fact, it was later discovered that Bright's disease is caused by a bacterium.) The way to cure diseases was to avoid eating 'foods that fight'. You should not mix proteins and carbohydrates in the same meal, and you should eat foods which restore the body's natural balance between acids and alkalis. There is no scientific evidence to support this theory whatsoever. The rules are rather complicated to observe and inherently contradictory, and the whole idea of food combining is nutritional nonsense. But in our faddy age the idea of food combining has caught on, and more than half a million copies of Thorsons paperbacks explaining it have been sold. The Hay Diet was given a particular boost when it was revealed in 1991 that the Duchess of York had been following it. It is possible to lose weight observing the regime because it greatly increases the intake of fruit and vegetables at the expense of more calorific foods. But there are profound problems with the general theory:

1. The idea that we need to go on a diet to 'detoxify' our bodies is absurd, though Dr Hay's diet is only one of many 'detox diets'. Besides nutrients in food there is a vast array of other substances which, if they were to accumulate in the body, would be toxic. Fortunately we are adequately equipped with mechanisms that enable us to break down and excrete these toxins so they don't accumulate. 'Detox diets' usually consist of fruit, raw vegetables, water and yoghurt but have little if any meat or fish. A low-calorie regime like this can lead to weight-loss. But such diets in general, and Dr Hay's in particular, are based on the misconception that fruit and raw vegetables are low in toxins and that meat and fish are high in them. In fact raw vegetables such as cabbage and onions are high in naturally occurring toxins whereas meat and fish are virtually devoid of them. Also, when the body takes in such natural toxins it can break them down and eliminate them more efficiently when on a high-protein diet provided by meat or fish.

2. Dr Hay's theory went on that acid wastes build up in our bodies and upset our acid/alkali balance. This is a misconception. A herbivore like a rabbit has alkaline urine, a carnivore such as man has acidic urine; but in both cases the body is constantly regulating the acid/alkali balance. For instance, our bodies produce alkali substances to eliminate the acidic by-products of digesting meat protein. Sodium bicarbonate (which is alkaline) neutralizes the sulphuric acid that is produced during the process. The acid/alkali balance in our bodies (known technically as the Acid Base Balance) is constantly maintained as part of a finely tuned mechanism. The idea that it gets 'upset' easily by the nature of the foods we eat is ridiculous.

3. Incompatible foods, such as carbohydrate and protein

should not be eaten together in the same meal – these, according to Dr Hay, are the 'foods that fight'. Observation of this rule, it is claimed, will improve digestion and absorption of food. This is nonsense. Almost all plant foods contain protein *and* carbohydrate. So how can you separate them? The basic staple foods of most civilizations – such as rice, wheat, oats and maize – all combine the two. Potatoes, too, contain starch (carbohydrate) and protein. Milk is a particular problem – it contains protein, carbohydrate and fat! We are also advised not to eat cereals (carbohydrate) with beans and pulses (protein). This is the absolute opposite of good nutrition. Cereals eaten with pulses (beans on toast, for example) provide high-quality protein for the body. This is very important for children, vegetarians and societies where little meat is eaten. So this part of Dr Hay's thesis is dangerous hogwash.

A specific diet book, based on Dr Hay's mistaken ideas, was published in 1993 and became the latest bestseller about food combining. *The Food Combining Diet* by Kathryn Marsden is as full of erroneous ideas about nutrition, as you would expect from a book based on an out-of-date theory:

1. **'Mix starches with proteins at the same meal and the digestive system won't know if it is functioning on acid foot or alkaline horseback.'**

   This is baffling. We digest starch and protein together at almost every meal we eat. Most basic foods contain both these nutrients. The whole digestive system contains balances throughout and is not adversely affected by what different sorts of food you may eat at the same time. Moreover, not everything has to be digested. We now know that some indigestible carbohydrates (fibre) keep the large bowel healthy.

2. **'Our hunter-gatherer ancestors certainly didn't indulge in the kind of mixed food fiasco we are familiar with today.'**

But, if health is the issue, their average life expectancy was 28; ours is almost three times as much.

3. **'Keep all fruits away from main meals.'**

This is a potentially harmful fad and contrary to current advice on healthy eating. We should all eat fruit every day. We are most likely to eat it at a meal-time. And so we should.

4. **'Avoid processed, refined foods.'**

Does this mean we should not eat bread or rice, both of which are processed?

5. **'Nor would I recommend artificial sweeteners. The latest research tells us that diet foods, slimmers' meals and low-calorie drinks which contain artificial sweeteners are likely to make weight-loss harder to achieve. It seems they can increase hunger pangs by disturbing blood glucose control and appetite . . .'**

This idea has been floated for some time, but we are afraid that it won't wash – there are no studies which have actually proved it.

6. **'You will see from the Food Combining Diet menus that the 24 hours from Friday evening's supper through Saturday breakfast and Saturday lunch are made up only of fresh salads and fruits, no fat and no heavy protein. These clean alkaline-forming foods are easy on the digestion and help to flush out accumulated toxins from the bloodstream.'**

This is laughable. There is no evidence that alkaline-forming foods are easier on the digestion, there are no accumulated toxins in the bloodstream, and they wouldn't be flushed out even if there were!

7. At various points Kathryn Marsden recommends liquorice as a sweet substitute, dandelion powder to bulk out coffee and linseeds for constipation. There is nothing dangerous about these in moderation, but the idea that they are natural and especially health-giving should be questioned. All contain more natural toxins than hamburgers, which we are told to avoid altogether.

Overall Verdict: Dr Hay's theories are discredited and unsubstantiated by modern science. Today's nutritional science shows Dr Hay to have been a crank. The book encourages faddy eating and perpetuates the myth that there are specific combinations of food that will help you either lose or gain weight.

The Rotation Diet

This book was heavily peddled in the newspapers about five years ago. It changes the level of calorie intake from week to week – from 600 per day to 900, to 1200 to 600 and so on. The theory is that with relatively low calorie diets (see p.122) the body's metabolic rate (the speed at which it burns off energy) falls so that when the dieter returns to normal eating the body needs fewer calories. The result is that (as Geoffrey Cannon put it in his book ten years ago) dieting makes you fat. The Rotation Diet claims to avoid this **'reduced metabolism'** by changing the calorie intake. We do not accept this theory:

1. You may lose weight, but it is because of the sometimes drastic reduction in calorie intake.
2. Six hundred calories a day is too low an intake at any time – such a drastic reduction, even for a week, could lead to the same problems that other low-calorie diets cause.

3.   Our metabolism is too sophisticated to be 'fooled' in
the way the book claims.

Overall Verdict: Bad science, unproven theories and too drastic
a reduction of calories. We do not recommend this diet.

Size 12 in 21 Days

One of the more recent bestsellers is *Size 12 in 21 Days* by
Judith Wills. This book fits into the diet book stereotype
fairly well. It is a diet-plus-exercise programme. There is a
photograph of the slim attractive author on the front cover,
and the copy on the back claims: **'*Size 12 in 21 Days* can
reduce your vital statistics by up to *2 dress sizes* in *just 3
weeks*. Much more than an ordinary weight-loss diet, its
unique formula promotes rapid but safe inch loss *exactly*
where you need it.'** Unique formula, rapid loss – we have
been here before.

1.   **'At the end of the first week you can weigh yourself;
you'll find a loss of 6 lbs (2.7 kg) on average . . . Days
8–14 . . . This week you will be on a steady 950
calories per day – all easy-to-prepare, delicious meals
that will help you to lose up to 5 lbs (2.3 kg) this
week . . .'**

For women this is too rapid. It is not healthy or
effective to lose weight this fast. Besides, much of the
loss in the first week will be just water rather than fat.

2.   **'The 21 day diet is not in any way a crash diet, nor a
fad diet. It is a healthy, low-fat diet and it is within
government healthy eating guidelines on every nutritional aspect.'**

This is incorrect. Days One and Two of the diet only
contain 600 calories. The Department of Health's

COMA report on Very Low Calorie Diets (see p.54) recommended that no-one should eat fewer than 800 calories a day. The protein intake at this stage of the diet is also lower than it should be.

3. **'You literally will be melting body fat from stomach, hips, bottom and thighs with the fat-burning routine – an easy yet effective, graded walking programme.'**

   This sounds wonderful but gives an exaggerated view of how much energy walking uses up. Even cycling for one hour only uses up around 300 calories. Walking energetically for half an hour (while undoubtedly doing you good) only burns off approximately 150 calories. That is equivalent to just 17 grams of fat. Exercise is not an effective method of losing weight, though it may help prevent weight-gain. But, in any case, when exercising energetically the body will use up carbohydrate before it burns off fat (and this particular diet is relatively high in carbohydrate).

4. On the subject of carbohydrates it is admitted that they convert themselves to energy in our bodies much more readily than do the fats: **'And they actually speed up your metabolic rate, helping you to lose weight more quickly than on most other diets . . .'** Again, this is incorrect. No specific foods can boost the metabolic rate although whole diet plans have been written claiming they can. Metabolism describes the way our bodies use up energy. There is a basic rate at which our body ticks over just to keep the heart and lungs going. It is simply wrong to claim specific foods or diets can help us burn calories faster, rather like putting your foot on the accelerator of a car. Carbohydrates do not boost our metabolic rate, as this book suggests.

5. Great claims are made for how the diet affects your body: whiter eyes, healthier gums and better, clearer

skin, all in twenty-one days. Longer term, we're told, our . . . '**hair may become glossier, nails grow stronger, and so on**'. This is all part of the process of making people on diets *feel* better whatever the reality. We should point out that no medical evidence for these claims is put forward.

Overall Verdict: The book encourages rapid weight-loss and exaggerates the amount of weight that can be safely lost. There is little if any evidence offered for the efficacy of the diet and exercises. Some of the claims are ill-founded. It implies that dieting is a healthy activity.

There are precious few diet books that encourage sensible weight-loss, ordered, healthy eating and that do not push any of the top ten myths we referred to earlier. The *F-Plan Diet*, which sold more than a million copies in the early 1980s, offered a thousand-calorie-a-day diet with a high level of fibre in it. The idea was that bulky fibre would make us feel full and decrease our desire to eat. (After a while our stomachs probably adjust to a bulkier diet and the importance of fibre is now considered to be only one part of the healthy eating message.) But it was a reasonable weight-loss programme with no bogus science. One more recent example is the *BBC Diet* by Dr Barry Lynch. But responsible, reliable diet books are few and far between. As long as the vogue for thinness persists and as long as the fashion industry perpetrates its weird version of the ideal woman we will continue to 'go on diets'. To satisfy this urge more and more diet books will appear, year by year, with new fads and novel gimmicks. We advise you not to buy them. But if you must here is our checklist by which to assess them. If they promise any of the following things, definitely do not buy them:

- rapid weight-loss (more than 1–2 lb a week)
- cures for 'cellulite'
- 'detoxification'
- spot-reductions of fat
- metabolism boosting
- food combining
- reliance on one particular food, such as carrots, grapefruit or pineapple

It may seem harsh to restrict yourself to what seems such a meagre weight-loss per week. But, as we shall explain later, gradual loss is both better for the body and easier to sustain. Not least because, if you adjust your eating pattern only marginally and over a reasonable period of time, you are already beginning to form new habits – ways of not eating more than you need. A rapid reduction of food, a sudden regime as offered by most diet books, is no help at all. It is not something you can continue with at the end of the diet period.

Dieting Can Damage Your Wealth

It is not only our health that is at risk from dieting. Many of the diet 'products' are very expensive, particularly when you consider that most are worthless. Many of us are fighting a never-ending battle with our weight in which the slimming industry plays the part of the arms dealer, fuelling the conflict.

We used the BBC's *That's Life* programme to recruit volunteers for a trial of some 'slimming cures'. The results were published in *The Lancet*. Five hundred overweight volunteers took part in the trial, all with their doctors' permission. They were randomly divided into eight groups to receive different treatments for six weeks. We realized that because the volunteers were being watched on television they were likely to change their diet spontaneously and lose some weight whatever treatment they were allocated. So we invented a neutral, placebo diet which consisted of eating half a carrot before the main meal. There's no reason why a carrot should make us lose weight – we chose the term 'carrot diet' because there have been popular diets like the 'banana diet' and the 'grapefruit diet' in the past (there's no reason why any individual food should make us lose weight). We didn't tell the viewers the carrot diet was a placebo until we announced the results. We decided before the trial that a treatment would be judged successful if the volunteers lost significantly more weight than those on the carrot diet. The other 'cures' were all actual products on sale at the time. Limmits are an example of 'meal replacements' where specially prepared foods (normally milkshakes or cereal bars) take the place of two meals a day (see p.45).

Table 1.5 (overleaf) shows how many kilograms the dieters lost over a six-week period on the various treatments. None of the magic cures for weight-loss we tested worked. In fact the Bai-Lin tea, which had been heavily promoted in one of the tabloid newspapers, turned out to be an ordinary Taiwanese semi-fermented tea. We will come back to that.

You will note how the WeightWatchers organization and Slimming Clubs came out of the test. These are relatively responsible organizations that do not commit the sins identified in our earlier checklist. They do not encourage rapid weight-loss and try to assess volunteers for how much weight they can safely lose. Meal replacements (biscuits in this case) came out of our survey satisfactorily, too, in that genuine weight-loss was achieved with them. But recently we assisted in a further investigation of the huge and growing meal-replacement market. The results were published in *Which* magazine in July 1993. Amongst the eleven meal-replacement plans analysed only one could offer evidence of long-term success (a crucial criterion). Nearly all encouraged rapid weight-loss and some products were as

Table I.5

WEIGHT LOSS IN OVERWEIGHT SUBJECTS AFTER SIX WEEKS OF TREATMENT

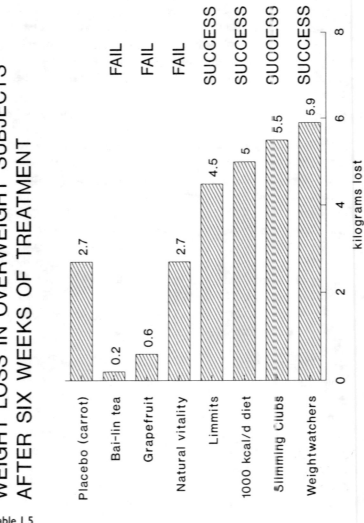

Sanders TAB, Woolfe R, Rantzen E (1990)
Lancet ii 918–920

high in sugar and calories as ordinary snack bars or milksha-kes (but more expensive).

Meal-replacement products are widely available over the counter in high-street shops, and are often manufactured by large food and drug companies. Such large companies apparently have no qualms about cashing in on the diet industry in this way. Few of the products help those buying them assess whether they need to lose weight. Only one brand we surveyed had a health warning on the packaging (Slim-Fast).

The idea for meal replacements grew out of the Very Low Calorie Diets (VLCDs) popular in the 1980s (see p.54). All you ate were special milkshakes and 'nutrition' bars. What meal replacements have done is adopt the principle of these liquid-formula diets, but only use it to supplant two of our three meals a day. In this way we consume fewer calories and lose weight.

There is now a draft European Community directive which attempts to control the claims and the formulation of meal replacements. It recommends that:

- products should not specify the amount of weight that can be lost
- products should state how rapid the weight-loss will be
- an individual meal replacement should provide at least 200 calories
- claims about feeling less hungry or satisfied should be banned

The draft also adopts declarations already required by Britain's food-labelling regulations: that products should state they work only as part of a calorie-controlled diet and that the shakes or biscuits should not replace all the meals in a day. It is not known when, or indeed whether, this directive will become law. But it provides a useful yardstick by which to judge the products.

Boots Shapers

There is either the Seven Day diet plan with milkshakes to replace two meals a day, or the Fruit and Fibre Five Day diet programme with two yoghurt shakes and a fruit and fibre bar per day. Most of the Shapers meals have fewer than 200 calories. And the yoghurt shake from the Five Day diet has only 99 calories. We also found that the Seven Day plan contained almost no fibre, whereas a healthy diet would contain around 18 grams of fibre a day. You would have to get all that from the one normal meal of the day. The Five Day diet has 8 grams of fibre in the bar. Lunchbars, that can be bought separately, are low in protein. If you relied on them as meal replacements, you would need to eat the equivalent of seven eggs in your normal meal in order to get the protein needed every day. These bars are now to be relabelled as part of Boots NutraSlim.

Boots NutraSlim

These are twelve-serving drums of milkshake mix. You have two shakes plus two 100-calorie snacks as well as an evening meal. This plan is better thought out than Shapers and provides adequate fibre and protein.

Carnation Slender

A choice of milkshakes and meal replacement bars. The shakes do not contain enough fibre, even in the new 'more fibre' recipe shakes. But the bar does have 6 grams of fibre.

Crunch & Slim

These are biscuits with which you can replace up to two of your daily meals. There is also a 'calorie-free' drink. Too rapid a weight-loss is promised: 'Lose up to 6 lbs in your first week . . . up to a stone in your first month.' They are too low in protein. From two Crunch & Slim meal replacements you would only get one-quarter of your daily protein requirement.

Fibre Slim

These shakes break food-labelling regulations. They claim to be 'low-calorie', and so a serving should contain fewer than 40 calories. In fact a serving contains 200 calories (in line with the EC directive). And even three servings of Fibre Slim still contain less than a third of our daily fibre requirement. So much for the name.

Firmaloss Seven Day Diet

This plan replaces your entire diet for a week with bars and instant meals at a cost of £17.99. The bars are not fortified, but a vitamin and mineral capsule is provided instead. Four of the instant meals are unappetizing-looking soups.

Firmaloss

A milkshake mix to replace one or two meals a day. It is low in some vitamins and minerals and fibre. The manufacturer of the two Firmaloss ranges plans to reformulate them.

Limmits

These are the biscuits from our earlier survey. You eat two cream-filled or muesli biscuits as a meal replacement once or twice a day. Four biscuits would give you 10 grams of fibre but, like Crunch & Slim, they are low in protein.

Slim-Fast

This is the most widely advertised product (you will be familiar with 'disc jockeys' and 'opera singers' endorsing it in joyous television advertisements). There are a variety of milkshakes, a fruitshake, soups and hot chocolate to replace breakfast, lunch and a snack each day. A 'nutrition bar' is an alternative for the snack. With 4 grams of fat, 12 grams of sugar and 110 calories per bar we think a healthier choice would be a piece of fruit. The soups are the best-balanced part of the range with a reasonable amount of fibre and much less sugar than the shakes.

The worst thing about Slim-Fast is its name and the claim that it is 'the healthy way to lose weight fast'. We believe there is no healthy way to lose weight fast.

Slim 'n' Trim

This five-day pack includes meal replacement bars, soups and a hot chocolate snack. If you are hungry during the five days, you are advised to eat extra vegetables. For the other two days of the week you are told to eat 'sensible low calorie meals'. Since Slim 'n' Trim is not fortified the claim that you can use it as long as you like is worrying. But the most bizarre element of Slim 'n' Trim is the 'amazing fat fighter capsule' which claims to help your metabolism convert fat into energy. No evidence is given for this. We think it is nonsense.

Overall Verdict: Meal replacements are big business, like diet books, because they promise rapid results. But they don't help us to learn to eat sensibly. Compared to an ordinary 1000-calorie-a-day diet they are a costly approach. Many are high in sugar or fat, particularly the biscuits. Few give proper advice as to what the all-important third meal of the day should be. They have the allure of being magic formulas but, in truth, these products are nothing of the kind. Sickly milkshakes and sweet biscuits hardly encourage any of us to eat more sensibly in the long run. In short, meal replacements are expensive sweets. We think they should all carry health warnings. (All the products were as described at the time of writing. They may have since been reformulated.)

Why not eat real food? By and large it is much cheaper, more nutritious and psychologically more rewarding. Here are some simple meals that provide about the same number of calories as meal replacements do:

- baked potato and cottage cheese
- poached egg and spinach on toast
- wholemeal roll filled with ham and tomato
- baked beans on toast, followed by an orange
- bowl of cereal and a banana

Any of the above are better for you and much more satisfying than a sickly chocolate bar or milkshake.

Healthy and Lean Options

Finally, a word or two about 'lean' or 'healthy' prepared meals. How lean or healthy are they? We compared sixteen beef lasagne products. Some were lean/healthy versions and some were their ordinary counterparts. The average energy value of those claiming to be healthy was 90 calories per 100 grams. But one of Tesco's Healthy Eating lasagnes had 110 calories per 100 grams while an Asda ordinary lasagne had only 106 calories per 100 grams. All had similar and relatively low fat contents – typically around 5 grams per 100 grams. Lean/healthy versions tended to have very slightly more sugar.

49

Overall Verdict: In general, eating 'healthy' or 'lean' prepared meals will not make a big difference to your diet.

Beyond Belief

As the cult of thinness has gradually perverted our view of our bodies, so a huge range of misleading and even fraudulent products has emerged to exploit the situation. Here we are not referring to books and meal replacements but to a range of pills, potions and magic cures. They don't help you lose body fat and we think pigs would fly before they ever did. Frequent claims are for 'rapid weight-loss', 'new medical breakthroughs' and 'moneyback guarantees'. Our A–Z of Dietspeak (see Chapter 7) lists the most common ones but here is a flavour of the delights available to you:

- *Slimming patches*. You attach a seaweed preparation to your skin and the claim is that it passes from the patch into your blood, speeding up your metabolism so you burn off calories faster. Nonsense.
- *Creams*. As we have pointed out, 'cellulite' was a word invented by the French cosmetics industry in order to sell creams. But rubbing in cream cannot remove fat deposits from the thighs. In October 1993 the Advertising Standards Authority asked the makers of Dior Svelte to withdraw national press advertisements for their product claiming 'This express action ultra-penetrating gel contains four plant extracts which have an unprecedented anti-cellulite activity'. The Authority concluded that evidence submitted by the manufacturers was inadequate to demonstrate that the product brought about an improvement of contouring through the elimination of fat.
- *Body wraps*. Believe it or not, some health farms and clinics are now offering to wrap people in bandages (a

sort of mummification) and cover them with mud. It is alleged that this opens the pores of the skin and the 'toxins' from around fat tissue come out. In fact weight-loss is achieved through loss of water (anyone would sweat trussed up like that). Any weight-loss or reduction in size is purely temporary. You can safely disbelieve anyone who uses the word 'toxin'.

● *Water-loss tablets*. Pills with a diuretic effect which make your body lose fluids. A number of herbs have this effect, and the process can fool you into thinking you've lost weight. One was advertised as follows: 'What a boon when you want to squeeze into your party dress and look and feel just right.' But any loss is temporary only and could be dangerous. Never take them.

● *Fibre and gel tablets*. The theory is that these swell in your stomach and make you less hungry. But, while having no effect on appetite, some could swell and block air passages in the throat or the intestines. The Government investigated and banned products with more than 15 per cent guar gum. Here are some other similar products which may not have been banned but whose claims for weight-loss are unsubstantiated:

Calorad: 'Lose weight without dieting – slim while you sleep . . . the simple theory behind Calorad's phenomenal success in the States and Canada is that by convincing your pituitary gland that essential nutrients are in steady supply . . . it will eventually work on all the body's faults – including excess fat.'

Slim-Line: Reported in the *News of the World* as a 'no diet cure for fatties'. An actor allegedly lost more than a stone in two weeks with tablets 'said to be made of totally natural ingredients which create a protective lining on the stomach, helping to trap weight-producing fats'.

Cal-ban 3000: '. . . the active ingredient comes from a 100 per cent natural plant source . . . when taken before mealtimes it bonds with the food you eat and "ties up" calories, preventing their absorption . . . a review of the customer files of this company revealed the names of hundreds of people who have lost up to 10 pounds the first week . . .' This was from an advertisement written in the style of a piece of editorial copy in a free magazine.

Speed-slim: Reported in the *Sunday Sport* (a journal even more reliable than the *News of the World*) as 'Miracle Slim Pills that Really Work . . . Speed-slim contains a Japanese herbal product, Galactomannan, that binds liquid in the stomach to prevent fat being absorbed . . . Speed-slim contains other herbal products which, when combined with water, fill the stomach to suppress appetite.' These pills were cautiously described in an advertisement elsewhere as 'an awesome discovery'. In fact they were just guar gum in another guise.

All these pills really offer is a unique combination of false science and genuine gobbledegook.

● *Grapefruit pills*. For a long time it was believed grapefruits helped you slim – that the acid in a grapefruit destroyed body fat. This is rubbish. It did not take long for a number of public benefactors to manufacture grapefruit pills. One example is Grapefruit 45: 'The Fat Burner Plan . . . apparently the Grapefruit 45 Fat Burner Plan is the secret which helps speed up the fat burning process.' The pills had no slimming effect but weight-loss might have occurred because they were sold with a diet plan.

● *Amino acid pills*. Slim-Nite pills claimed that you could 'Shape up while you sleep!' and 'research has proven that a certain combination of amino acids, taken before you go to sleep really does help you slim'. Amino acids are the basic building-block of proteins, and when protein is digested the body breaks it down into these acids for absorption. There is no evidence that, sold as a supplement, amino acids will help you lose weight. One brand of amino acid pills contained contaminated tryptophan (an amino acid used as a health supplement) and led to several deaths in the United States.

- *Teas.* As attractive as magic pills was the idea that by sipping tea you could lose weight.

Bai Lin Tea: 'Bye Bye Fat, buy Bai Lin.' This product, endorsed by page-three girl Samantha Fox, turned out to be no more than a fermented tea imported from Taiwan. 'I lost 7 lb without having to diet!' said the advertisement, and they even published a certificate of test results from the 'National Taiwan University'. But as we saw in our survey, it failed a controlled experiment. Its suppliers were subsequently prosecuted.

SINZ-ZI: Another slimming tea. Here they tried a novel scheme and sought '1000 persons' to participate in tests on the tea. They were lucky enough to be offered 110 days' worth for £29.95 (normal price £60). Another advertisement quoted Chinese Professor Zhang Shun-Yi ('I created a revolution') and claimed that the slimming tea affects body metabolism and the burning of fat cells. But tea cannot help you slim.

- *Negative calories.* A 'top selling' American book revealed '19 foods that cause you to lose weight'. It went on: 'Cakes? Cookies? Ice Cream? Yes! Continue to eat the foods you now enjoy. Just add 25% of the 19 foods to your regular meals. The "Negative Calories" contained in them will burn off the excess calories in bread, butter, even rich desserts.' We think this is a good comedy script.

Overall verdict: The simple truth is that to lose weight you have to take in fewer calories. Pills and potions such as these have nothing to do with it. They are often peddled in advertisements that are written to look like independent editorial material. Genuine articles trumpeting the arriving medical breakthroughs are not all they seem, either. Never believe any claims for slimming products and never, ever buy them. They will certainly damage your wealth and, in some cases, could damage your health, too.

Half Starved

There is one form of meal replacement which we would particularly urge you to avoid: Very Low Calorie Diets or VLCDs. They were a crash diet producing extremely rapid weight-loss which became popular in the early 1980s. They were supposed to provide all the nutrients you need except calories and usually in the form of a milkshake powder. But when several people died who were taking VLCDs in the United States great concern was expressed as to their safety.

The Department of Health's 'COMA' committee investigated Very Low Calorie Diets and in 1988 recommended that they should never have fewer than 400 calories for women and 500 for men in a day's supply. COMA advised all dieters to try less drastic diets, emphasized the maximum period of four weeks and stressed that children, the elderly and pregnant women should never use VLCDs at all. What worried COMA was the risk that rapid weight-loss (more than 4½ pounds a week) might mean losing more than just water and body fat. When semi-starved the body starts to attack 'lean' tissue as well, such as muscles. The heart is a muscle, and the particular worry was that VLCDs could lead to cardiac problems. (In Michigan health experts were so concerned that they issued a statement detailing a number of potential complications including heart problems, dehydration, hypoglycaemia, hair-loss, anaemia and emotional problems.)

The other major concern about VLCDs is that some of our bodies adapt themselves to the drastically lower calorie intake by reducing their metabolic rates. So when dieters return to normal eating the body no longer needs as many calories as it did before the diet. It stores the excess as fat. In other words, VLCDs might make you *put on weight* in the long run.

A survey of *Which* readers (all of whom were 'slimmers') found that one in six had tried VLCDs. All had lost weight and most professed themselves satisfied. But when questioned further it emerged that almost two-thirds had not kept the weight off.

Today Very Low Calorie Diets, reformulated as they may have been, are seen by most experts as a treatment for extreme obesity only, to be used under supervision in hospital and only if the obesity is more of a threat to life than the VLCD would be. But not all obesity specialists agree with this. Professor John Garrow of St Bartholomew's Hospital believes there are no circumstances in which they are justified. He believes that even severely obese patients can still lose weight on a conventional diet. Worse, he believes VLCDs undermine the faith obese people should have in conventional diets. Their confidence in their ability eventually to regulate their own eating is unnecessarily destroyed.

Our Verdict: Very Low Calorie Diets should only ever be used under medical supervision as a treatment for extreme obesity, where life is threatened. They should never be used by people who are plump or slightly overweight or who merely desire to look thinner. They carry the risk of both physical and psychological side-effects.

Clinically Dangerous

More hazardous than VLCDs, more exploitative than any of the diet potions we have exposed, is the trade in slimming drugs. These include amphetamines and related drugs which act on the central nervous system as appetite suppressants. They are sometimes prescribed by doctors to clinically obese people to help them lose weight However, many of these drugs are potentially addictive and can have nasty side-effects such as headaches, insomnia and even hallucinations. Common brands are called Duromine, Tenuate Dospan, Apisate and Ionamin. The data sheets issued by the manufacturers of these drugs confirm that they are only for treatment of the obese. As controlled medicines they can only be prescribed by a doctor, though they can be legally dispensed by others.

We assisted in an investigation for BBC's *Food and Drink* of six 'slimming clinics' in the London area. These are private clinics where people who want to lose weight can go and can see a doctor. At all these clinics researchers of ours, of normal weight, were prescribed amphetamine derivatives. And the sad fact is that, as we write, a similar survey has found that slimming clinics are still handing out these hazardous drugs to people who are neither obese nor need to lose weight at all.

Later we explain 'Body Mass Index' (BMI), a method of working out whether we are underweight, normal, overweight or obese (see Chapter 3). But for the purpose of our investigation you need to know the following:

Researcher One   BMI 21.2   Normal
Researcher Two   BMI 23.3   Normal
Researcher Three BMI 27.0   Overweight (but not obese)

First we sent them to two non-medical slimming operations. At a WeightWatchers slimming club all three were given advice based on calorie-controlled diets and gradual weight-loss. At a Nutri System clinic (no longer operating in Britain) all three were given similar advice. However, the picture at six specialist clinics was very different and very disturbing.

Knightsbridge Diet Clinic: Researcher One was told by the doctor she didn't really need appetite suppressants, but when she pressed for them she got them. She was later rung by the clinic and reminded to come back next week having taken the pills. On her return visit she was told to make sure she took the pills. This was our researcher with the lowest BMI, someone who was slim and didn't need to lose any weight at all. Researcher Two was told he could lose a stone in three weeks and given slimming pills. When he returned a week later not having lost weight (he, of course, had not taken the pills) the clinic owner dispensed more drugs, double the strength of the first prescription. The clinic owner was not medically qualified.

Our third researcher was given pills on both visits, again at double strength the second time. She was overweight but not obese and therefore the drugs were never designed for her.

National Slimming Centre: All three researchers were prescribed suppressants on both visits. Researcher Two was told not to mix alcohol with the drugs. On the way out he was given a free 'goodie' bag. Inside were Martini miniatures.

Medical Slimming Services: Researcher One was refused slimming pills and told they were only for people with a lot of weight to lose. Strange, because Researcher Two (who hadn't any weight to lose) was given a week's supply of suppressants. On his second visit, when he said he wanted to lose a stone, they gave him a double-strength prescription.

London Slimming Centre: All three researchers were prescribed slimming pills and on one occasion they were dispensed by someone other than a doctor. Here Researcher One was erroneously measured at a stone over her real weight.

Just Slim Clinic: All three researchers were prescribed pills on both their visits.

Diet Consultation Centre: Researcher One was refused pills but Researchers Two and Three were given suppressants at both visits.

We wondered how thin people had to be before these clinics would refuse slimming drugs. So we sent four more volunteers to the London Slimming Centre. All four were really slim, at the bottom end of the normal range of weight. But two were told they could lose weight and one was even given suppressants. (We have faithfully recorded what we found at the clinics during our survey – their practices may have changed since.)

What can we say about clinics that make profits out of people's misery and neurosis over their weight? What can we say about qualified doctors who prescribe drugs to people of normal weight? Let us merely quote a suppressant manufacturer and two medical experts. Dr Harry Massheder, who works for Merrell Dow, makers of Tenuate, said: 'It's outrageous and reprehensible that normal weight patients have been prescribed them.' And Dr Nick Finer, the obesity expert at the Luton and Dunstable Hospital, said this about the four volunteers sent to the London Slimming Centre: 'These people were thin. They were either at the low end of the normal weight or thin. And again, I mean these people had no weight problem . . . bizarre.' Professor Paul Turner is a clinical pharmacologist at St Bartholomew's Hospital and chairman of the Government's Committee on Toxicology. He put the whole seedy business into perspective: 'Overweightness . . . really needs to be properly investigated either through the general practitioner or through a hospital. If the patient is worried about their weight, but he's not overweight are they anorexic? Do they suffer from this condition – anorexia nervosa – that has its own problems? Now to give a patient with anorexia nervosa a drug that has central stimulant properties or that would be harmful to them seems to me to be very foolish.'

Overall Verdict: *Never* attend a private slimming clinic or take amphetamine-related drugs without referral from your GP. Always seek the help of your GP and get referred, if necessary, to a reputable obesity specialist.

The Unkindest Cut of All

Appalling though it may sound, in the 1970s surgeons began to experiment with cutting fat away from the body of people who wanted to be thinner. Not only was this cosmetic surgery very painful, but also healing problems were suffered by the patients (though perhaps *victims* would be a better word). Then in the early 1980s liposuction was developed in France: a thin tube (a 'canula') is inserted under the skin to suck out the fat. The procedure gained a good deal of publicity when Michael Caine was reported as having had it done in order to slim down for a film part. The irony is that younger people, who may only want a little fat removed and whose skins are still relatively elastic, can be pleased with the results. Older people in their forties and fifties, who more often request the operation, can be left with flabby sagging skin because it is no longer elastic and able to spring back into a more youthful position. The operation is quite traumatic and represents a risk:

- blood clots (i.e. thrombosis)
- permanent numbness can result in the area
- severe bruising for several weeks
- loss of blood
- lowered immunity to infection

It is normally performed under general anaesthetic, which can itself traumatize the body. Diabetics run a higher risk of infection afterwards and people with high blood pressure should never have the operation.

Overall Verdict: Liposuction is a highly profitable operation to carry out. Anyone offering liposuction should be a fellow of the Royal College of Surgeons and, preferably, a member of the British Association of Plastic Surgeons. But our verdict is that the operation is never necessary and the side-effects are not worth the alleged 'benefits'. We need to eat sensibly and accept the basic shape of our body, not cut bits off it.

At every stage the diet racket is evil and exploitative. Every one of the billion pounds we spend annually is paid for by ill health and unhappiness. We buy our daughters dolls that give them a completely distorted view of what a normal, feminine body should look like. We reinforce this bizarre image with painfully thin 'stereotypes' on almost every fashion page (they are, in fact, anything but stereotypes). Many of the models who present this image are themselves very sick individuals. We smoke cigarettes as slimming aids even though they lead to heart disease and cancer. We accept a series of fantasies in a whole range of diet books in our pursuit of the cult of thinness. We flock to buy rip-off pills with magic formulas and we eat expensive 'meal replacements' full of fat and sugar while ignoring real food – all to fit a false image of ourselves. We go on life-threatening diets, and some even take slimming drugs in order to achieve the perfect body. And does it ever work? Does any of these nostrums make us either slim or happy? In the short term, perhaps they do; in the long term, never. A government survey published in 1991 showed the confusion there is about dieting. Some men and women who claimed they were on a diet in fact had calorie intakes higher than people who were not dieting!

Meanwhile the incidence of eating disorders climbs inexorably, particularly amongst young people whose lives, at their age, should be healthy and full of optimism. This is a sick society and it is getting sicker all the time. Is there any way of curing this growing malaise? A sensible attitude to food and a healthy scepticism towards the diet industry would be a start. That is what this book seeks to promote. Thankfully there are others banging the same drum. The year 1993 saw a growing anti-diet sentiment crystallize into formal campaigns both here and in the United States. In Britain, Mary Evans Young has set up Diet Breakers. She says dieting has reached epidemic proportions and is now a Western version of Chinese foot-binding – in other words, dieting is institutionalized torture of women's bodies. Mary runs courses at which she explains in graphic terms how diets do not work, how skinniness is not healthy and how, in order to be attractive, you do not need to resemble an Oxfam advertisement (it is a sick reflection that Western dieters, in a land of plenty, spend much of their waking life trying to resemble the starvation victims of the Third World where food is not available). Mary Evans Young has organized 'No Diet Day' complete with a motion in the House of Commons. And she campaigns tirelessly against advertising such as the mail-order catalogue that classifies 36 or 38 inch hips as 'large'.

Diet Breakers want to see the dangers of dieting declared on all slimming products. They want to see the fraudulent pills and the diets that don't work more systematically exposed and challenged in the courts. And, perhaps most important of all, they want to see information put into all schools to counter the propaganda of the fashion and diet industries. Think of the effort and resources put into the AIDS health campaigns. Think how many more this problem affects.

Not long ago *Slimming* magazine asked its readers why they most wanted to diet. These were the top five reasons:

To look better	26%
For health	21%
To feel better	17%
To wear nice clothes	13%
To restore confidence	11%

Only one of the five was specifically about health, the other four were by and large about fashion. We now need to alter our view of fashion. We need clothes for women that adorn their bodies, not desecrate them. We need to face the fact that, as the diet industry expands, so do our waistlines. As a nation we are getting fatter all the time. Dieting does not work. *Dieting is not the solution. Dieting is the problem.*

Eating normally, and with pleasure not guilt, does not have to lead to weight-gain. To change our view of food and of our bodies we need to understand why we eat what we eat. Why is food, like sex, the source of such neurosis? Why does it involve guilt and pleasure in equal measure? Chapter 2 explains how our attitudes to food are formed.

2 WHY DO WE EAT WHAT WE EAT?

We have already looked at how obsessive and wrong-headed we can be about food, particularly when aided and abetted by the diet industry. One defence against developing these harmful attitudes is to understand what our natural instincts towards food are. So in this chapter we get back to basics and discover why we eat what we eat.

At the turn of the century, Sigmund Freud blamed the sexual taboos prevalent in Austria for the neurotic attitudes seen in society. Food now rivals sex as a neurotic focus in our culture. We have become obsessed by body shape and food. Food is also blamed for many psychological problems such as bedwetting and hyperactivity in children, and for adult health problems such as heart disease and cancer. Eating certain foods now seems threatening. Many of us have developed this unhealthy attitude towards food and we are in danger of losing the pleasure that can be derived from eating. Where did we go wrong? In this chapter we explain the factors that now affect our choice of food and regulate our appetites.

Cyril Connolly remarked that inside every fat man there is a thin one trying to get out. But it is not only overweight people who have eating disorders – underweight people have them too. On the one hand, there is an ever-increasing proportion of people becoming obese and failing to lose weight. Yet at the other end of the scale many people who do not need to lose weight are trying to and often succeeding. This is responsible for the increased prevalence of eating disorders associated with dieting such as bulimia and compulsive eating. Perhaps inside every thin person there is a fat one trying to get out.

Our national neurosis about dieting mainly affects young

women. Middle-aged men and post-menopausal women, who are the ones that should be most concerned about being overweight, tend to ignore all dietary advice. We found that 95 per cent of people attending a commercial slimming clinic were women and their average age was about 35. When we carried out our slimming trial for *That's Life* (see p.42), 75 per cent of the volunteers were women.

In order to indicate how neurotic some women are becoming about food here is a selection of typical statements made by women with eating disorders:

● I am always reading articles and books about dieting
● I buy diet products
● I have gone on eating binges
● I feel extremely guilty after eating
● I am preoccupied with food and the desire to be thin
● I avoid eating when I am hungry
● I feel that food controls my life

A MORI survey carried out in July 1993 found that one in four women is so worried about food that she doesn't enjoy eating. Our perception of food has become so distorted that one cynic remarked foods can now be divided into just four groups:

● Good for you but tastes bad (e.g. boiled fish, potatoes, brown rice, bran, skimmed milk, salads)
● Bad for you but tastes good (e.g. butter, bacon, cheese)
● Makes you fat and ugly (e.g. lard, pork pies, Scotch eggs)
● Eat it and die (e.g. cream cakes, chocolate, premium ice-cream)

But there is no such thing as good or bad food – there are just good and bad diets. What matters is the relative contribution each food makes to the diet and how much you eat in total.

Nutritionists have traditionally divided foods up into five

food groups: dairy produce; meat and fish; fruit and vegetables; fats; and cereals and starchy foods. The basis of this division was that you need to include foods from each group to achieve a balanced diet. This has now been replaced with a food pyramid (Figure 2.1 overleaf) which puts emphasis on the relative amounts of each food that should be eaten with emphasis on the starchy foods and cereals and fruit and vegetables nearer the bottom and less on meat and fish, dairy foods and fats nearer the top.

Unfortunately our general attitude to food and dietary choice is a long way from this sensible, ordered model. A myriad of other factors, many quite irrational, affect our eating patterns. In all societies food has a symbolic role, often related to primitive beliefs. Human beings have a strong tendency to believe in magic, and there are a large number of food taboos, mainly affecting women and children, that are a product of superstition. In parts of Africa children are forbidden to eat eggs because it is believed that if they do they will turn into thieves. In Indonesia it is taboo to give young women big bananas. In some developing countries tinned baby-milks are believed to be superior to breast milk. Closer to home, some people believe that drinking milk causes catarrh. None of this is true. And of course, in our society, many people believe that there are magic combinations of food that will make you lose weight. People from Africa or Asia might well think it strange that British people believe they can only lose weight by living on a diet of expensive diet-milkshake powders and snack bars!

Food also functions as a status symbol, like serving caviar at a party, or as a sign of friendship, like giving a box of chocolates to your neighbour. People will eat the caviare or the chocolates not necessarily because they're peckish, but because they've learned that doing so is one of the rules of social etiquette. We would be offended if our neighbours

THE BRITISH HEALTHY EATING PYRAMID

A GUIDE TO CHOOSING A HEALTHY DIET

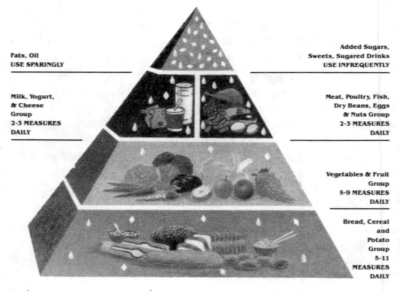

Fats, Oil
USE SPARINGLY

Added Sugars,
Sweets, Sugared Drinks
USE INFREQUENTLY

Milk, Yogurt,
& Cheese
Group
2-3 MEASURES
DAILY

Meat, Poultry, Fish,
Dry Beans, Eggs
& Nuts Group
2-3 MEASURES
DAILY

Vegetables & Fruit
Group
5-9 MEASURES
DAILY

Bread, Cereal
and
Potato
Group
5-11
MEASURES
DAILY

KEY ◐ Fat (naturally occurring and added) ◇ Sugars (added)   These symbols show fats, oils and added sugars in foods.

Each day choose foods from all five groups.

Eat most of the large bread/cereal group at the bottom.

Eat least of the small fat and sugar group at the top.

A measure is a small portion, or a unit of food (eg slice of bread, piece of fruit).

Young, active, not overweight: Eat the larger numbers of measures shown.

Older, inactive, overweight: Eat the smaller numbers of measures shown.

Produced by the Flour Advisory Bureau and the Dunn Nutrition Centre

Figure 2.1

refused to accept chocolates because they didn't feel like sweets at the time.

We eat to live. Food is essential to life. Some people (usually thin moralizing types) argue that as long as we only eat *from need and not from greed* (that is, we only eat when we are hungry) then we would not over-eat and get fat. But, as we shall see, it is not as simple as that. Our desire to eat is determined by a complex interplay of biological signals from our body along with learned patterns of behaviour. Hunger and appetite (the desire to eat) are controlled by chemical signals that tell us that we are hungry. When we are infants these dominate what we eat. To the infant, milk also provides comfort and security. So from an early age the desire to eat becomes imbued with other meanings. But it is sparked off by one of the most fundamental instincts. It determines why we eat when we eat.

Basic Instincts

We are born with instincts that tell us when we need food. For example, a newborn baby will automatically cry and suckle when hungry. The human body is equipped with sensors that detect when fuel supplies are low and more food is required. An empty stomach or a low blood-sugar level triggers the signals that tell us we are hungry. These biological signals make us feel hungry and increase our appetite. After having eaten the signals change. Our stomach is full and the blood-sugar level rises. This is when we say we are full. The technical term is *satiety*.

We feel full for different reasons. Our appetite for a single food will decrease the more we eat of it. But our appetite for other foods remains about the same. Most parents are aware of how childen eat only half of their main meal and say that they are full up but amazingly can find room for pudding.

This means that more will be eaten when a meal contains a variety of foods than when it contains just one. It is why single-food diets (e.g. banana or grapefruit diets) and the Hay Diet (which forbids certain combinations of foods) may decrease calorie intake but at the same time torture our taste buds. They frustrate our instinct for variety. They also lead to a nutritionally unbalanced diet because only by choosing a range of foods can we get all the nutrients we need. As we shall see, it is only when there is virtually unlimited choice that our taste for variety gets the better of us.

We derive immense pleasure from eating. From an early age we learn to choose foods because we like them, not because we know their nutritional value. The newborn baby has an innate preference for sweet foods and a dislike for bitter tasting ones. This is also linked to our bodies' need for nutrients. Human beings, unlike most other animals, require vitamin C in their diets. Primitive man would have depended on eating fruit, which is also sweet, for a supply of vitamin C. Sugars and starches, which are broken down into sugars in the gut, are rapidly absorbed into the blood-stream. Between twenty and thirty minutes after eating sugar, the level of blood-sugar (glucose) rises rapidly and triggers sensors in the brain that suppress appetite. One slimming product with the unfortunate name of AYDSLIM consists of fudge-like cubes which are high in glucose. It is claimed that eating these cubes prior to a meal will dull your appetite making you eat less. Indeed, Dr John Blundell at the University of Leeds has indeed shown that subjects given a sugary drink about half an hour before lunch do eat marginally less at the meal. But in the long run, there is little evidence that products like AYDSLIM are of value in controlling appetite, especially in the obese.

In fact, there is evidence to the contrary. Dr Barbara Rolls of John Hopkins University, Baltimore, has carried out a large amount of research on the factors controlling satiety.

She looked to see if sweet foods affected appetite and she also substituted artificial sweeteners for sugar in some of her tests. She concluded that sweetness did not influence appetite. Other factors clearly do, though.

Fit to Burst

We gave volunteers different breakfasts containing the same amount of food energy (calories), protein and fibre but varying amounts of fat and carbohydrate. We found that subjects struggled to get through a high-carbohydrate low-fat breakfast compared with a high-fat low-carbohydrate breakfast.

The high-carbohydrate breakfast contained a lot of sugar and was quite bulky:

> Coco-Pops
> Honey
> Sugar
> Bread
> Low-fat spread
> Orange juice
> Skimmed milk
> Scrambled egg
> Lean bacon

whereas the high-fat breakfast slid down a treat:

> Sausages
> Bacon
> Fried bread
> Fried egg
> Fried tomatoes
> Full cream milk

Barbara Rolls agrees that the bulk of food eaten in a meal is the main factor determining how full we feel. So there is little doubt that bulky diets (such as the F-Plan Diet) decrease appetite in the short term. However, in the longer term we get used to the increased bulk and adapt by eating more.

One of the reasons we find it easier to eat fatty foods than starchy ones is that they are less bulky. Carbohydrates also get into the blood more quickly and affect our appetite after about half an hour. After eating a fatty meal, by contrast, there is a delay of about two to three hours before the newly absorbed fat is present in the blood. This is too late to tell us we are full and to stop eating. So although, gram for gram, fat has more than twice the calories of carbohydrates, it takes much longer for it to make us feel we've eaten enough.

Civilizing Influences

As society has developed so has our attitude towards food. Some of the developments have been civilizing, some not so. Early man was a hunter-gatherer and his food supply was restricted by his ability to catch and harvest food. Man then learned to cultivate cereals and other crops, to domesticate animals and to fish. This allowed more time to be spent on other activities besides foraging for food, and so civilizations flourished. The supply of food was often limited and unpredictable so that food shortages were common, as they still are today in many developing countries. Obesity is uncommon in developing countries for these reasons. But in developed countries the supply of food is so abundant and diverse that it no longer restricts what we eat. Not only do we have a bountiful food supply, but also a huge variety and much of it in a form that is convenient to eat. The sheer variety of food on offer in British supermarkets brings tears to the eyes of visitors from Eastern Europe.

Most natural foods require preparation to make them palatable. Only a few natural foods can be eaten as they are, such as fruit and nuts. Cereals such as wheat, oats and rice have to be processed and cooked before they can be eaten. Beans need to be cooked for up to an hour and a half. In the past, the resources to process foods were also limited, and this and the drudgery of food preparation restricted access to food ready to eat. Compare this to the present time where it is possible to conjure up something to eat in a few minutes, to grab something to eat from the fridge or just to graze on fast food in any high street. This change is a consequence of large-scale food processing, convenience foods and the variety of gadgets (microwaves, food processors) available in most people's kitchens. This means at home we are exposed to more food in a form that can be readily consumed than ever before. It is well known that over-exposure to food and drink increases intake – this is why cooks are more likely to be fat and publicans more likely to be alcoholics.

There has been a phenomenal growth in the popularity of fast food. Back in the 1860s, fish and chips was an important addition to the monotonous diet of town-dwellers. It offered a cheap and nutritious meal to ordinary working people. It was popular because it was convenient – an important factor as many people didn't have proper cooking facilities. But now fish-and-chip shops have been joined by fried chicken, pizzas, hamburgers, baked potatoes, doughnuts and ethnic foods (Chinese, Indian and Greek takeaways). One only has to look at the transformation of the major railway stations in Britain. In the 1970s there was typically a station bar and a sit-down restaurant selling soggy fish and chips and sad cheese-and-tomato sandwiches. Now there is a profusion of fast food outlets such French bread shops, croissanteries, burger bars and pizzerias. Most shopping centres and supermarkets also offer a tempting array of takeaway food.

There is little doubt that this diversity of food makes eating more fun. But it is also this constant exposure to food that makes it difficult to resist over-eating.

Convenience foods have also resulted in a loss of cooking skills in the population. Generations are now growing up who no longer know how to prepare or to cook food from raw ingredients. This means that they generally eat convenience foods and so, once they become adults, they will be particularly prone to eat more than their bodies need.

The food industry has also capitalized on our desire to nibble and munch with an awesome variety of snack foods, most of which are high in fat and calories. Snack foods by definition are those that can be consumed instantly, usually standing up or on the move. Snack foods have always been popular with children and they probably play an important role in helping them meet their high energy requirements. But many adults will graze on snacks and nibbles if they are on offer. As the comedienne Victoria Wood remarked, food eaten standing up doesn't count when you are on a diet. But there is nothing inherently wrong with snack foods; it is again our attitude towards them that is at fault.

The food industry spends millions of pounds on finding out what makes a product popular. If the customer doesn't like the food, then it won't sell. But this is only part of the story. Research shows that most consumers say they favour 'healthy eating'. However, the evidence is that they only pay lip service to healthy eating while actually voting with their forks – taste, quality and convenience are what really count. The food industry is constantly looking for new markets and consumers, and one way is to exploit this ambivalent attitude to health. Diet drinks such as Diet Coke and Diet Pepsi playing on our fear of sugar as a wicked food rapidly expanded the soft-drink market. Perhaps one of the most successful marketing transitions in recent years, lying at the other end of the spectrum, is the 'naughty-but-nice' foods. The development of frozen confectionery has to be admired as a wonderful piece of lateral thinking. First Mars launched the Mars ice-cream bar and now it has been joined by most of the other famous brands of chocolate bar. Frozen and chilled desserts have been one of the fastest-growing sectors in the food market. They are convenient, they taste good and they sell. Later we explore this apparent contradiction between the popularity of diet drinks with a healthy profile and the high sales of wicked, frozen confectionery.

The Eye of the Beholder

It is often said that we eat with our eyes. The way food is presented is another factor affecting our choice. In chic restaurants dishes are designed to be elegant as well as appetizing with terrines looking like William Morris wallpaper. The colour as well as the appearance of food affects our choice. We have become accustomed to expect foods to be certain colours. For example, the British expect peas to be bright green. In fact processed peas go a dull grey-green colour. In response to consumer scares about food additives, several manufacturers tried selling tinned peas without their added colour, but they were unpopular. Colour preferences vary between countries and are associated with what we recognize as food. For example, the British expect butter to be bright yellow whereas on the Continent butter is pale yellow. In the United States they expect egg yolks to be pale yellow, but in Britain we expect them to be dark orange. And it has been observed that children like eating foods that are bright orange (carrots, fish fingers) while they dislike dark green foods (cabbage, spinach).

Some years ago Dr Ralph Watson at the University of London carried out an interesting study to see how colour affected our food choice. The subjects of the study were asked to select different foods from a buffet, and the researchers recorded their preferences. In subsequent weeks the same subjects were asked to make their choice from the same array of foods that had been dyed a variety of different colours such as red, pink, blue, green and purple. They found that they tended to avoid blue and purple foods. And some subjects thought they were drinking chocolate when they were given coffee dyed red. Thus even the appearance of food can confuse our basic instincts.

Hurry, While Stocks Last

Advertising has a great influence on what we eat. Advertising on children's television is dominated by adverts for soft drinks, breakfast cereals and confectionery. Characters are created that appeal to children. For example, Ronald McDonald, Tony Tiger and the Milky Bar Kid. There is little doubt that children's preferences for food are affected by advertising. Most parents have been pressured by their children to buy a particular brand of soft drink or cereal (which they often refuse to eat after extracting the free plastic dinosaur from the packet).

The food industry, like the tobacco industry, sometimes argues that advertising only influences the choice of brand rather than the type of product consumed. We don't agree with this. Advertising is the main means by which consumers get to learn about diet products. A few years ago, adverts for slimming products were confined to free magazines. This has now changed. Untested and potentially unsafe diet products are widely advertised in the national press. We are bombarded with junk mail offering phoney diet products and have stickers placed on our cars asking us to enrol in diet programmes. Television advertising plays an important part in the unhealthy growth of the meal-replacement market (e.g. Slim-Fast) and undermines our faith in ordinary food.

Advertising experts recognize that eating represents a combination of pleasure and balance. By pleasure they mean giving in to temptation, indulgence and sharing an experience with family or friends. By balance they mean recognizing aspirations for health and appearance. Advertisements for food products commonly appear alongside features on how to use them or the health benefits they offer. Currently there are many advertisements for 'lite' or 'fat-reduced' products. Market research suggests consumers perceive three main benefits from these types of product:

- slimness (therefore attractiveness)
- health (priding themselves on a rational choice)
- freedom from guilt

However, consumers often find that lite/fat-reduced products take some of the pleasure out of eating. By contrast advertising for Häagen-Das high-fat ice-cream uses 'wicked', sexy and indulgent images. The result is that we are encouraged to use lite or fat-reduced products as a trade-off against the 'wicked products'. Tesco's leaflet extolling the virtues of its 5 per cent fat spread had this to say: 'If you are already on a diet which is overall low in fat and there is no need to cut down on calories then by replacing butter with Lowest Ever you can treat yourself to a generous ½ ounce (16 g) serving of clotted cream and still be saving 2 g fat.'

It is known that the fatter people are, the less sugar they consume and the more likely they are to use artificial sweeteners and low-fat products. There is nothing wrong with low-fat products and artificial sweeteners if they are used sensibly. But we seem to believe that by using an artificial sweetener or drinking diet cola it gives us licence to eat something 'forbidden' and high in calories such as a bag of nuts or a bar of chocolate. So instead of eating rationally we are now tending to veer between two extremes. We have only ourselves to blame for our peculiar attitudes.

Advertising on television aimed at women is more concerned with shape and seductiveness, and is dominated by images of slenderness. But luxury items such as chocolate and premium ice-cream are also targeted at women. As a consequence, certain foods can acquire negative or threatening meanings. For example, many women associate tasty foods like chocolate and chips with gaining weight. This is linked to fears about losing their attractiveness. Consequently, eating these foods makes them feel guilty. This is a completely unbalanced approach to food which has been aided and abetted by the food advertisers. It is a combination of extremes which is as foolish as the 'yo-yo' diets we looked at in Chapter 1. But guilt about healthy eating and the desire to indulge ourselves are only two weapons in the advertisers' arsenal. There are others.

I'm In with the In-Crowd

Advertising has become increasingly sophisticated. For example, the Nescafé advertisement depicting the subliminally sexual relationship between a power woman and her male neighbour, who is always dropping in to borrow some coffee, was so popular that the relationship was used for a bestselling book, *Love over Gold*. By consuming a certain food you are permitted to share in an experience or belong to a select group. Thus you are what you eat and drink. One can see similar patterns in other age groups. Ice-cream bars in the shape of Mickey Mouse (cutely known as 'rat bars' to the staff at Disneyworld) appeal to young children because they perceive it as sharing in a slice of Disney. And burger bars with names like Planet Hollywood or Hard Rock Café offer teenagers a hunk of Hollywood.

Advertising of food and drink has moved into the sports arena, formerly dominated by the tobacco industry. Many of the great sporting events are sponsored by food and drink companies, and sports personalities receive large amounts of money for endorsing food products. Most of this advertising is aimed at men rather than at women. Food companies are trying to neutralize bad publicity and to cultivate a healthy image to go with their product. For example, Coca-Cola, which is very sugary and could therefore be perceived as unhealthy, has sponsored many of the Olympics. Lucozade Sport is another sugary drink promoted by an Olympic gold medal winner. Mars boosted its image by sponsoring the London Marathon, much to the chagrin of health educators who have often griped at the Mars advertising jingle, 'A Mars a day helps you work, rest and play'. And McDonald's are the sponsors of the 1994 football World Cup. There is nothing intrinsically wrong with Mars bars or McDonald's, by the way, but many people who are seriously overweight or suffer from eating disorders openly admit to eating them in excess.

Forbidden Fruit

English food was once feared throughout the world because it was so monotonous and poorly cooked. Yet in recent years there has been a huge growth of interest in cooking and food preparation, and we have seen a renaissance of good food and drink. This is highlighted by the proliferation of television programmes and magazines about food and the increased variety of foods available. It is a paradox that we are now as equally obsessed with dieting and weight control as with titillating our taste buds.

As a nation we are becoming promiscuous with our palates seeking out new food experiences (much like the different sexual positions in the *Kama Sutra*). The term *gastroporn* has been used to describe the tantalizing dishes displayed in magazines that are thumbed through and salivated over like top-shelf girlie magazines – look but don't touch. You could call it culinary masturbation. Terms like 'naughty but nice' encourage us to indulge. Like the sexual revolution of the sixties, the food revolution of the nineties brings with it complex sentiments. There seems to be an unwritten rule in Anglo-Saxon countries that states that if you enjoy something it must be bad for you.

In fact our enjoyment of food is often tempered by guilt. But illicit acts give a certain *frisson* to life. As a child, the mother of one of the authors would climb over the wall of an orchard in a nearby farm and scrump apples. The scrumped apples, she recalled, tasted out of this world. But then the farmer, who presumably saw her scrambling over the wall, told her father that she could help herself to apples whenever she wanted. The apples were no longer forbidden fruit and didn't taste the same. The symbolism of food and guilt goes right back to Adam and Eve. Food is like sex – it brings guilt and pleasure in equal measure.

As we mentioned, each society has its own set of beliefs about food. The French eat horses and the Chinese cook dogs. Dogs and horses as a food are taboo in Britain. Some eating patterns are strongly interwoven with religious belief. For example, pork is forbidden to Muslims and Jews. Christianity depicts gluttony as one of the Seven Deadly Sins. Yet in other religions obesity is associated with the gods themselves. For example, Buddha and the Egyptian god Osiris are both depicted as fat. But the puritan ethic still has a pervasive influence on Anglo-Saxon culture. Religious writings talk about abstaining from pleasures of the flesh, fasting and self-denial. Baden Powell (founder of the Boy Scout movement) in his book *Scouting for Boys* had this to say about rich food and self-abuse: 'Sometimes the desire is brought on by eating food that is too rich, or sleeping in too warm a bed with too many blankets. It helps at times such as these to take a cold bath or shower or exercising the upper part of the body by arm exercises, boxing etc.' He also had this to say about getting up early: 'A scout trains himself to the habit of getting up early. When once in the habit it is no trouble at all to him, as it is to some fat fellows who lie asleep after daylight has come.' The puritanical ethic dictated that food should only be consumed for sustenance, not for pleasure – much as the belief that sex should only be for procreation. It also suggested that fat people were automatically lazy and debauched.

The food reform movement, with its origins in the middle of the last century, was also dominated by puritans such as Quakers, Seventh Day Adventists and Salvationists. They zealously promoted the conflicting messages of prohibition and guilt. Foods which were regarded as stimulants such as alcohol, tea, coffee and spices were forbidden along with meats, which was believed to give rise to lusty thoughts. To this day many food reform groups are dominated by killjoys.

You Are What You Eat

An attack on our food is often seen as an attack on our culture. Vegetarians refuse to eat meat and fish, and vegans avoid all food of animal origin. The Conservative politician John Gummer has been slugging it out with these men of lettuce saying that vegetarianism is an attack on Christian values. What you choose to eat may also be a political statement. You may not have bought fruit from South Africa because you are an opponent of apartheid. If you buy organic food, for example, it may be because you are concerned about the environment. You may buy free-range eggs because you think that battery farming is barbaric. There are so many reasons one can give for not eating food.

Eating has an important socializing function. Imagine a child's birthday party without a cake or a wedding reception without alcohol. We also use foods to punish and to reward.

As we grow up we acquire a lot of emotional luggage from food that can be a burden in later life. We learn to associate certain foods with both pleasant and unpleasant sensations or events. Some people feel guilty or sick when they eat certain foods. This can result from the association of an unpleasant event with a particular food. Eating that food on future occasions causes unpleasant memories to flood back. One of the authors vividly remembers a boy at school forced to finish his tomatoes so that he developed a total phobia of this innocent fruit. The very sight of tomatoes physically nauseated his body from then on.

Traditionally families would eat together. This social function is particularly strong in Jewish culture where the preparation of food and eating together helped maintain their cultural identity. The pattern of eating was until recently relatively structured for all of us with defined eating occasions such as breakfast, lunch and dinner. Social changes that have occurred mean we eat together far less frequently. There has been a breakdown in the whole culture of formal meals. This is illustrated by the massive growth of takeaway foods and eating out. Female emancipation also means that the stereotypical role of the woman as cook and housekeeper has declined (but, where it happens, women still bear the brunt of the shopping and cooking). It is now not uncommon for members of a family to eat different foods at different times. This breakdown in structured eating, along with the increased opportunities to eat, is crucial in understanding why we are losing control over what we eat. If it is socially acceptable to eat whenever you like, and the food is constantly available, then it makes ordered eating increasingly unlikely. Particularly when other motives come into play.

We often eat for comfort, as George Orwell put it in *The Road to Wigan Pier*: 'When you are unemployed, which is to say you are underfed, harassed, bored and miserable, you don't want to eat dull wholesome food. You want to have something a little bit "tasty".' For many people, sweet food represents comfort and security. Think how often we eat sweets, not because we're hungry but because sweets taste nice and make us feel better. Some people become compulsive eaters. For example, Mary Evans Young (who runs the anti-diet campaign Diet Breakers) admits she would binge on five Mars bars at a time. She also prepared and ate separate meals from the rest of her family before she recognized she was a compulsive eater.

It can be seen that what we choose to eat is often not determined by our body's need for food but by patterns of behaviour learned from childhood and carried into adult life. We learn to associate certain foods with pleasure or a certain lifestyle. Eating and drinking are an integral part of our social life, and, above all else, are to be enjoyed and not feared. As we have shown, there are no particular foods that make us fat; it is our attitude towards food that is wrong. We are reluctant to accept responsibility for our actions, particularly when they bring us pleasure. Our attitudes to fatness and body shape are also important. In the next chapter we look at how they and dieting affect our health.

Whether you are consciously aware of it or not, you, too, have your own menu of food meanings and responses, and this influences the kind of diet you eat. Answering the following couple of questions *honestly* will help you confront this aspect of your appetite.

Q1 Just supposing . . .

A There's something tasty in the fridge. Would you go and finish it off? *('Well, it's a shame to let it go to waste'.)*

Frequently [ ]   Occasionally [ ]   Never [ ]

B You're on an aeroplane and the stewardess puts one of those meals in a plastic tray in front of you. Would you polish off the lot even if you weren't hungry? *('What the hell, it's free, isn't it?')*

Frequently [ ]   Occasionally [ ]   Never [ ]

C You're preparing a meal. Would you nibble as you go along? *('One for the pot and one for me and one for the pot and . . .')*

Frequently [ ]   Occasionally [ ]   Never [ ]

D You've had a row with your partner or boss. Would you take it out on the biscuit tin?

Frequently [ ]   Occasionally [ ]   Never [ ]

E It's late at night and you're alone with the telly. Would you nibble away at something to console yourself?

Frequently [ ]   Occasionally [ ]   Never [ ]

Count up the number of times you chose 'frequently', 'occasionally', or 'never' for Question 1. Which response did you choose *most often*?

Frequently. Deep down inside you know you're something of a food junky – just the sight of food turns you on and when things go wrong you crave your food-fix. You're not necessarily very overweight, but if you don't wean yourself off this habit of comfort-eating, you might end up that way – which isn't very healthy and might make you rather more unhappy.

Occasionally. You're human and you can get tempted to eat when you're not hungry – but if your other answers were 'nevers' then, by and large, you've got your appetite under control. No real harm in indulging your whims once in a while. But remember the tendency to temptation is there and try not to get hooked.

Never. You rarely yield to food unless you're hungry and you don't use it as an emotional prop. On the face of it, this is a healthy attitude. But before you congratulate yourself prematurely, check your rating for the second question.

Q2 Decline or fall?

A Do you try to eat less at meal-times than you'd really like to?

Frequently [ ]   Occasionally [ ]   Never [ ]

B When offered food or drink, do you turn it down because you're worried about your weight?

Frequently [ ]   Occasionally [ ]   Never [ ]

C Do you make a point of choosing lower-calorie meals?

Frequently [ ]   Occasionally [ ]   Never [ ]

Count up the number of times you chose 'frequently', 'occasionally', or 'never' for Question 2. Which response did you choose *most often*?

Before we analyse your answers to this question, there is one more thing we need to know. Would a doctor say you were seriously overweight?

If you are not seriously overweight and you mostly answered *Frequently*: You treat life like a permanent slimming diet, don't you? There's no need to keep such a tight hold of your intake. Letting go doesn't mean you'll be sunk by the fatty you fear within. Regain a more balanced attitude to food by eating when you are hungry and you will find the scales steady themselves. Select from a range of foods, too – there's no such thing as bad foods, only bad diets.

If you are seriously overweight and you mostly answered *Frequently*: Well done. You're taking positive action; but make sure you're eating sensibly, though, and not starving yourself in your desire to lose weight too quickly.

Occasionally or Never: If you're comfortable that way, so be it. But you may be storing up problems for yourself.

3   IN FATNESS AND IN HEALTH

We are beset on the one hand by the diet racketeers and on the other by advertisers and lifestyles that encourage unnatural patterns of eating. *Fatness, plumpness, overweight, obesity* – these are dirty words. Whinge as we may about the twin tyrannies of fashion and the slimming industry, is it not true that anyone who isn't slim threatens their health? This is indeed the received wisdom, but it is simply wrong. In this chapter we examine how plump people are actually healthier than skinny ones. We begin by exploring something that really is unhealthy: our attitude towards weight.

The Weight Problem

The constant pressure on women to pursue a slender image has led them into a continuous cycle of weight-loss followed by weight-gain – the 'yo-yo' diet trap. Slim 'good' looks are now seen as an essential part of a woman's sexual identity. Recent surveys show that more than a third of women are dissatisfied with their shape. Many typically complain that their bottoms or hips are too big. The lack of fashion clothes in appropriate sizes is one reason for their dissatisfaction. We have seen how the bulk of women's clothes, particularly the latest designs, are made several sizes smaller than that of the average woman. Consequently, women are pressurized to lose weight. To be fashionable they have to be able to squeeze into an under-sized dress.

Men are more likely to be proud to be plump. Success, power and money are often most important to men's egos. They prefer a well-fed opulent look to fashionable slimness. But a MORI poll published in July, 1993 found that men are becoming more concerned about their shape. For example, many men find it offensive to be greeted with the remark, 'Oh, you've put on weight,' and take the remark, 'Oh, you've lost weight,' as a compliment. The survey found that young men are more likely to be concerned about their shape and, unlike older men, want to have a muscular physique as well. So men now feel pressurized to 'go on a diet' as well as women. Dr Jane Usher, a psychologist at Guy's Hospital, fears that men are being led into the diet trap by women who are already ensnared. Both men and women are now made to worry about their shape and size because of comments from others – most commonly from their partners.

In the last chapter we highlighted how neurotic our attitude towards eating has become. But we have become similarly neurotic about our shapes. Here are some remarks commonly made by women:

- Being naked, such as taking a bath, makes me feel fat
- I have imagined cutting off the fleshy areas of my body
- I feel excessively large and rounded
- I am worried about my flesh being dimply
- I feel ashamed of my body
- I am preoccupied with the thought of having fat on my body
- I am worried about other people seeing rolls of flesh around my waist or stomach
- I have not gone out to a social occasion (e.g. a party) because I feel bad about my shape
- I am preoccupied with the desire to be thin

Figure 3.1 shows the results of some research carried out by Nasira Sheik at King's College, London. She asked young women to look at different body shapes shown below – from A (emaciated) to L (very fat). The young women were asked the following two questions:

1 After looking at all the shapes, which of the outlines do you think resembles your figure?
2 Rate the shapes on how appealing you think they are.

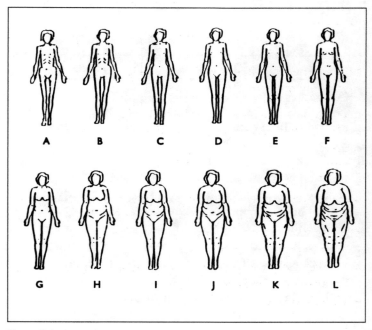

Figure 3.1

Here is what the results showed:

SHAPE	1. Which shape they thought resembled their figures	2. Which shape they thought most appealing
C	6%	–
D	8%	9%
E	22%	34%
F	34%	56%
G	23%	1%
H	5%	–

Table 3.1

In answer to question 1, most of the women saw themselves between E, F and G – size F being the average. This is, indeed, what you expect for young women – sizes E, F and G are quite normal.

In answer to question 2, most thought that body shape F was ideal but many preferred the leaner shapes D and E. In contrast only 1 per cent thought body shape G was ideal.

What can we conclude from this? Many young women want to be slimmer than they are. In doing so they are often seeking a shape that is leaner than is physiologically normal. That, in reality, is the chief weight problem facing us today. But the great irony is that other research reveals that this perfect shape women want to achieve is actually slimmer than the ideal most men find attractive. Most men prefer shapes F, G and H whereas, as we have seen, most women prefer D, E and F. Shapes D and E are, in fact, less attractive to men because they seem less feminine and more androgynous. So the pressure of the fashion and diet industries has led many young women to desire a body shape for themselves that:

- is slimmer than the norm for women of their age
- has no health advantages
- is less attractive to men

Attitudes towards body shape aren't just concerned with fashion and sexual attractiveness, though. They also spill over into how we treat people. The 'gravitationally challenged' are discriminated against at school and at work. Fat children are teased, and many employers are reluctant to employ fat women. For example, some supermarkets would not employ women who were fat, and a US airline was sued for applying weight restrictions to their flight attendants (they then relented and allowed them to be a little plumper). In Singapore (a country that takes public health issues so seriously that people are heavily fined for not flushing public loos and hanged for possessing drugs) all conscripts to the army are also given an acceptable weight. The time it takes them to get down to this approved weight is added on to their national service.

Until relatively recently, fictional characters who were fat were not always portrayed in a bad light – they could be seen as jolly, cheerful and kind, but perhaps feckless, like Falstaff, Mr Pickwick or Billy Bunter. Nowadays, many films portray fat people in a stereotypical way as ugly, greedy, immoral, stupid, slothful and villainous. Even in squeaky clean, politically correct America the villain in the film *Jurassic Park* is portrayed as a fat slob – he is untidy, greedy and living on a diet of junk food. It does, however, still seem acceptable for comedians to be fat or plump: for example, the American soap star Roseanne or British comics such as Dawn French, Mel Smith or Robby Coltrane. Discriminating against people because of their shape is just as reprehensible as discrimination on the grounds of race, religion or gender.

But so strong is the anti-fat influence in society that such behaviour remains acceptable.

A hundred years ago it was different. To look lean and gaunt was associated with poverty and tuberculosis, while plump curvaceous women were not only acceptable, they were desired and thus portrayed by painters of pornographic pictures. To look 'well nourished' was considered admirable. Thinness is still regarded as unattractive in many countries. In African, Middle Eastern and Asian cultures, fatness is still regarded as sexy as it was here in the Victorian era. Fatness is also regarded as a sign of fertility (and, as we shall see, underweight women can indeed be barren). In Asia the gaudy film posters usually display *svelte* Western film stars as plumper than they really are – the artists put a stone or two on them as a matter of course.

Body Shape

Our body shape is mainly determined by our body build and not by what we eat. People fall into three categories:

- Ectomorphs – body shape determined by their skeleton. They are typically tall, thin and delicate.
- Mesomorphs – body shape determined by muscles. Well built, like many sports players.
- Endomorphs – body shape determined by fat. Typically rounded shape, tapering at the extremities.

Our shape is believed to be determined during early development. We are born one of these three shapes, and there is nothing we can do to alter our body build. Body build is largely inherited, although recent research by Professor David Barker at the MRC Epidemiology Unit in Southampton suggests that it may also be influenced by how well we grow in our mother's womb. We need to recognize that we naturally come in all shapes and sizes.

Unfortunately, body build and shape have been confused with fatness. For example, fashion currently favours an ectomorphic body (thin and delicate). But a mesomorph or endomorph simply cannot be transformed into an ectomorph by diet.

Women are naturally fatter than men, and their fat is predominantly on the buttocks and thighs (pear-shaped). Men are leaner and have a more muscular build than women, but when they lay down fat they do it on the upper part of the body (apple- or barrel-shaped). Roughly 18–30 per cent of the weight of a healthy woman is fat whereas in men it is only 12–20 per cent. This female fat plays a very important role in reproduction. A certain threshold level of body fat, somewhere between 15 per cent and 18 per cent, is necessary for fertility and expression of secondary sexual characteristics (development of breasts and suppression of hair growth on the limbs and face). This is because body fat, along with the ovaries, is involved in making the sex hormone oestrogen. Oestrogen is responsible for the pear-shaped fat deposits on the hips and thighs of women.

If a woman's level of body fat drops below about 15 per cent then monthly periods will stop because not enough oestrogen is being produced. This commonly occurs in ballet dancers and female athletes who are too lean. It can also result in the growth of facial hair. Reproductive function is normal in women with 18–30 per cent body fat because they can produce enough oestrogen. But, if the amount of body fat is very high, excessive amounts of oestrogen are produced, and this can also cause monthly periods to stop. It can also increase the risk of endometriosis (inflammation of the lining of the womb) and skin problems. But the key thing is that a certain amount of body fat is essential to maintain the production of oestrogen within normal limits. The relatively high level of fat in women is nature's way of ensuring that reproduction does not occur unless there is a sufficient energy store to cover the energy cost of pregnancy. You would never learn how natural and valuable female fat is from the fashion or slimming industries. By promoting super-thinness they are literally anti-feminine.

Female fat has other benefits. The hormone oestrogen helps protect women from heart disease and osteoporosis (brittle bones). Heart disease is linked to high levels of blood cholesterol. Oestrogen helps keep blood-cholesterol levels down by increasing the capacity of the liver to remove cholesterol from the bloodstream. This is almost certainly why heart attacks are rare in women prior to the menopause. Oestrogen also helps prevent the loss of minerals such as calcium from the bones. Such loss leads to osteoporosis which is a major cause of fractures of the leg and hip in the elderly. In fact more women die from the consequences of osteoporosis than from breast cancer. Fat and plump women are much less at risk of osteoporosis than skinny women. After the menopause, oestrogen levels fall and women change their fat distribution to that of the male pattern and their risk of heart disease greatly increases. Hormone replacement therapy, which involves giving oestrogen, reverses this change.

How Fat Is 'Fat'?

Obesity is a technical term used by doctors, but it has taken on a very negative connotation. It actually means excessive deposition of fat. But what is that in practice? Obesity is usually measured in terms of weight and height. Put in simple terms, if you are obese you are too short for your weight. There are tables that give desirable ranges of weight for height. Various cut-off points are used to define excess weight. *Overweight* is usually defined as 10–19 per cent greater than optimal weight and *obesity* as being in excess of

20 per cent. *Underweight* is usually defined as more than 10 per cent below the optimal weight.

The term *optimal* or *desirable weight* is often used by doctors and the slimming business. But how were these figures derived? Who says what the optimum is? Life insurance companies record the weights and heights of people when they take out policies and calculate the odds of having to pay out early according to an individual's weight for height. The desirable or optimal weights are based on those weights for height that are associated with the least likelihood of early death and therefore the lowest risk to the insurance companies. Insurance policies are predominantly taken out by men in their twenties and thirties, and very few of them die before they are 50. The insurance companies' main concern is having to pay out for early deaths. Early on they found that very fat men are more likely to die suddenly under the age of 40 years so they weighted their premiums accordingly. However, this definition of desirable weight is too simplistic. As we shall see later on, the relationship between obesity and longevity is different. It can also be argued that people who take out insurance policies may not be typical of the general population because many sick individuals are excluded from cover. While, from an actuarial point of view, the insurance companies got it right, their desirable weights for young men have been extrapolated to older men where the relationship between weight for height and risk of death is different. Weight at age 25 is rarely the same as weight at age 40. Most men get fatter as they get older, so it is really not appropriate to make a health judgement about the weight of a 45-year-old man based on the same criteria as for a man in his early twenties. Desirable weights for women are based on even shakier assumptions, as we shall see later on.

Measuring body weight for height is an indirect measure of obesity as it is assumed that increased body weight is due to increased fat. This is not always the case. The density of fat is less than that of water, whereas muscle is more dense. Individuals who have developed their muscles from athletic training are generally heavy for their height but not fat. The United States Army realized this in the days of conscription where very overweight men were rejected for military service. They found that they were rejecting recruits with a Rambo-like body build. Body building and wrestling are now greatly in vogue. A 6 foot 4 inch wrestler typically weighs 280-300 pounds and on the figures alone would be defined as obese, but obviously he is not.

In view of all these problems, distortions and over-simplifications, optimum or desirable weights have now been replaced with ranges of acceptable weights. These allow for changes in weight with age and cover both men and women in broad categories (Table 3.2).

Acceptable weights for men and women

Height		19–34 years		35 years +	
feet & inches	metres	lbs	kgs	lbs	kgs
5'0"	1.52	97–128	44–58	108–138	49–63
5'1"	1.55	101–132	46–60	111–143	50–65
5'2"	1.57	104–137	47–62	115–148	52–67
5'3"	1.60	107–141	49–64	119–152	54–69
5'4"	1.63	111–146	51–66	122-157	55–72
5'5"	1.65	114–150	52–68	126–162	57–74
5'6"	1.68	118–155	54–71	130–167	59–76
5'7"	1.70	121–160	55–72	134–172	61–78
5'8"	1.73	125–164	57–75	138–178	63–81
5'9"	1.75	129–169	58–77	142–183	64–83
5'10"	1.78	132–174	60–79	146–188	67–86
5'11"	1.80	136–179	62–81	151–194	68–88
6'0"	1.83	140–184	64–84	155–199	70–90
6'1"	1.85	144–189	65–86	159–205	72–92
6'2"	1.88	148–195	67–89	164–210	74–95

Source: USDA 1991 Dietary Guidelines for Americans
Table 3.2

Many slimming clinics and diet products still set people target weights based on ideal weights instead of on these acceptable weights. This is a wicked practice that helps sell their products and services to people who do not need them.

Body weight is a relatively good index of obesity only if it is related to height. The French mathematician, Quételet, invented an index to express weight for height, and this is commonly called the body mass index (BMI) or Quételet index. BMI is the method most often used to classify obesity in adults. It is calculated by dividing the weight in kilograms by the height in metres squared. For example, a man who is 85 kilograms (13 stone 4 pounds) would divide that by his height of 1.72 metres (5 feet 8 inches) squared and come up with a BMI of 28.7.

Calculate your BMI

Body Mass Index = the ratio of body weight divided by height squared

$$BMI = \frac{\text{Weight in Kilograms}}{(\text{Height in Metres})^2} \quad \text{or} \quad \frac{W}{H^2}$$

Example 1:
Male: weight = 85.0 kg, Height = 171.5 cm = 1.72 m

$$BMI = \frac{85.0}{(1.72)^2} = \frac{85.0}{2.96} = 28.7$$

Example 2:
Female: weight = 65.0 kg, Height = 165.0 cm = 1.65 m

$$BMI = \frac{65.0}{(1.65)^2} = \frac{65.0}{2.72} = 23.8$$

Table 3.3

Body Mass Index Table

(kg/m²)

Height (inches)	19	20	21	22	23	24	25	26	27	28	29	30	35	40
						Body weight (pounds)								
58	91	96	100	105	110	115	119	124	129	134	138	143	167	191
59	94	99	104	109	114	119	124	128	133	138	143	148	173	198
60	97	102	107	112	118	123	128	133	138	143	148	153	179	204
61	100	106	111	116	122	127	132	137	143	148	153	158	185	211
62	104	109	115	120	126	131	136	142	147	153	158	164	191	218
63	107	113	118	124	130	135	141	146	152	158	163	169	197	225
64	110	116	122	128	134	140	145	151	157	163	169	174	204	232
65	114	120	126	132	138	144	150	156	162	168	174	180	210	240
66	118	124	130	136	142	148	155	161	167	173	179	186	216	247
67	121	127	134	140	146	153	159	166	172	178	185	191	223	255
68	125	131	138	144	151	158	164	171	177	184	190	197	230	262
69	128	135	142	149	155	162	169	176	182	189	196	203	236	270
70	132	139	146	153	160	167	174	181	188	195	202	207	243	278
71	136	143	150	157	165	172	179	186	193	200	208	215	250	286
72	140	147	154	162	169	177	184	191	199	206	213	221	258	294
73	144	151	159	166	174	182	189	197	204	212	219	227	265	302
74	148	155	163	171	179	186	194	202	210	218	225	233	272	311
75	152	160	168	176	184	192	200	208	216	224	232	240	279	319
76	156	164	172	180	189	197	205	213	221	230	238	246	287	328

Source: NIH (US)

Table 3.4

There is a quicker way off calculating your BMI by using table 3.4. Find the appropriate height in the left-hand column. Move across the row to a given weight. The number at the top of the column is the body mass index for the height and weight. Each entry gives the body weight in pounds for a person of a given height and body mass index. Pounds have been rounded off.

It is easy to calculate your body mass index. But you can use the nomogram shown in Figure 3.2 to see which category you fall into.

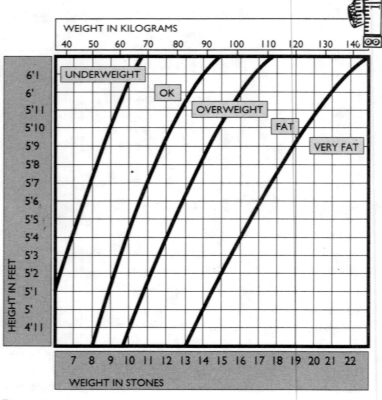

Figure 3.2

The term *morbidly obese* is used by doctors to describe obesity that seriously threatens health. The body mass index, it should be noted, is *not* suitable for assessing whether children are overweight as their relationship of weight to height differs. With children one has to take into account their stage of maturation. **No child should ever be placed on a diet unless a doctor orders it.**

The ratio between waist and hip is another quite good measure of fat distribution. The ratio should be less than 0.95 (apple-shaped) in men and in women less than 0.8 (pear-shaped). The higher the ratio the more fat there is in the abdomen. From a health point of view this is undesirable whatever your body mass index. Some men are pear-shaped and some women apple-shaped. To measure the ratio, measure your waist circumference (not omitting your tummy) and your hip circumference. Divide the waist measurement by the hip measurement to get the waist–hip ratio. For example: waist 34 inches and hips 40 inches.

$$\text{Waist–hip ratio} = \frac{34}{40} = 0.85$$

Fatness and Health – How Big a Hazard Is It?

Contrary to popular belief, body fat in itself is not a sign of unhealthiness. Women are twice as fat as men yet they live four to five years longer on average. We can judge the health risks of obesity by asking these two questions:

- Does it shorten life?
- Does it increase the risk of disability?

We need to recognize that immortality is not an alternative. Longevity in itself is not a good goal if quality of life is poor. As they age, human beings develop a number of debilitating conditions that decrease quality of life. Doctors use the term *morbidity* to describe the presence of these non-life-threatening disorders, such as arthritis and skin complaints. The aim is to stay fit and active for as long as possible. Ideally, perhaps, we should be like bumble bees that busily fly along and then one day suddenly drop dead. There is something to be said for a fatal heart attack, especially if it occurs at a ripe old age.

The risk of developing medical disorders such as diabetes, high blood pressure and gout increases with increasing body weight. The rate of increase of risk is slight until the body mass index exceeds about 28 and then it increases rapidly. So the risk is greatest in those who are very fat. It is unusual for an individual with a body mass index of greater than 40 not to have a medical condition associated with excess weight, and so doctors describe this condition as *morbidly obese*. Being extremely fat at a young age certainly increases the risk of sudden death from heart disease in both men and women. On the other hand, the health risks of being underweight are as great and often greater than being morbidly obese. In contrast plumpness has positive benefits for health, particularly for younger women. Not only do they live longer, but also they are less likely to suffer from several common complaints.

In men, plumpness may have adverse effects on health, especially if their fat is concentrated in the abdomen. The term 'Syndrome X' is used to describe the metabolic disorder that is characterized by impaired glucose tolerance, gout, raised blood pressure and blood cholesterol commonly seen in middle-aged men with pot bellies. Syndrome X is strongly associated with a greatly increased risk of heart disease. Many men with Syndrome X would not be regarded as fat but have an unhealthy distribution of body fat. Their health certainly benefits if they lose their pot bellies by taking regular exercise and eating sensibly: their blood pressure and blood-cholesterol levels fall and their glucose tolerance improves.

While there are some advantages to plumpness, extreme fatness is as undesirable as being extremely underweight. The health risks of underweight and overweight can be ranked accordingly using the body mass index:

BMI	RISK
Less than 18	Very high risk
18–20	Moderate risk
20–25	Average risk
25–30	Low risk
30–35	Moderate risk
35–40	High risk
40	Very high risk

Table 3.5

We are constantly bombarded with information about the health risks of obesity. *The Health of the Nation*, the Government's first attempt at a comprehensive health policy, aims to reduce the prevalence of obesity from its current level of 13–16 per cent to less than 6 per cent. But not everyone agrees that obesity or fatness is such a big health problem. According to Dr G. V. Mann: 'Obesity has been wrongly indicted as a major health problem . . . This evil view of obesity has come from four places: the insurance industry, the medical moralizers (usually themselves thin), the drug industry, and the docile, unquestioning nutritionists who are too often dupes of the faddists and the hucksters.'

In the public's mind obesity is often linked to an increased risk of heart disease both in men and in women. However, most experts do not regard obesity on its own as an independent risk factor for heart disease in the absence of raised blood pressure, raised blood cholesterol or diabetes. But doctors generally agree that if you have medical conditions such as

101

raised blood pressure, cholesterol or diabetes, then it is important to keep your weight under control.

Ancel Keys, who masterminded the famous 'Seven Countries Study' which looked at the relationship between lifestyle factors and heart disease, concluded that fatness did not influence longevity or risk of heart disease when other factors such as blood pressure and blood-cholesterol levels were taken into account. He found, for example, that Mediterranean Italians were fatter than the Finns, but that the Finns were much more likely to die from heart disease. He said: 'No study has reported a direct linear relation between relative weight and mortality.'

Why is there confusion over the importance of obesity and health? Besides the statistics from the insurance companies, there are a number of studies where heights and weights were measured in young men and women and the subjects were followed up over a period of sixty to seventy years to see how long they survived and what they died from. Very few of these subjects were obese when they were young and so what these studies show is a relationship between body build and health rather than between fatness and health. Table 3.6 shows the survival rates in men.

BMI	Percentage men failing to survive to age ...						Category
	20–29	30–39	40–49	50–59	60–69	70–79	
18–19	0	0.2	3.6	9.6	24.3	50.8	Lean
21–22	0	0.9	3.3	8.1	19.9	38.4	Average
24–25	0	1.1	3.5	8.3	18.0	35.1	Optimal
32–33	0	1.7	5.1	11.2	22.8	41.0	Obese

Source: The 1979 Build Study

Table 3.6

Young men who had a low body mass index of 18 were more likely to die of cancer, but as the body mass index increased risk of heart disease increased and that of cancer fell. Life-expectancy was lowest in the men with the lowest body mass index and highest in those in the group that were in the mid-range to plump group. The death rate under 40 was highest in the fattest group, but overall their life-expectancy was still greater than the leanest men.

There is good evidence that men who maintain their weight do not show the same age-related increases in blood pressure and blood cholesterol. However, most adults gain weight with ageing. Being overweight as a 40-year-old man slightly increases the risk of dying prematurely but after the age of 50 men who are overweight live longer than those who are underweight. One explanation for the longer life-spans of fatter 50 year olds may be that some of the thinner 50 year olds are smokers. By this age their habit is beginning to take its toll. The risk of dying from smoking is very much greater than the risk of dying from being even seriously overweight.

There has been a huge increase in the prevalence of obesity among British men, from 6 per cent in 1980 to 13 per cent in 1991. But rates of heart disease have fallen by about 30–35 per cent over the same time period. If obesity was a major factor in causing heart disease, then one would expect to see rates rising.

Table 3.7 shows the survival rates in women according to body mass index.

BMI	Percentage women failing to survive to age ...							Category
	25	35	45	55	65	75	85	
< 18	0	1.0	3.4	11.9	27.7	50.9	78.4	Underweight
18–20	0	0.5	1.9	6.8	18.0	38.2	71.3	Lean
20–22	0	0.5	1.8	4.9	12.8	32.8	67.9	Average
26–28	0	0.3	1.6	4.4	11.5	30.5	65.3	Plump
34–36	0	1.0	2.8	6.8	16.5	38.9	72.1	Obese

Source: The Norway Study
Table 3.7.

For women there is no specific relationship between body mass index and death rates. This applies to all diseases including cancer and coronary heart disease. But women who could be described as plump live the longest. You won't hear that fact from the diet industry – they need to keep it as quiet as possible.

Heart attacks are extremely rare in women prior to the menopause, and obesity or plumpness in women prior to the menopause is not associated with increased risk of heart disease. In fact the opposite is true: thin women are more likely to have an early menopause and therefore lose their protection from heart disease. Anorectic women who allow their body-fat levels to fall very low have very high blood-cholesterol levels, which increases their risk of heart disease (if they haven't already died from starvation first). After the menopause, there is a change in fat patterning and obesity. This is strongly linked to increased risk of heart disease. Heart disease is the main cause of death in women after the menopause, and women are more likely to suffer from angina (chest pain) than men. Most of the deaths from heart disease in women occur at a relatively old age. The preva-lence of obesity almost doubles after the menopause. It is known that hormone replacement therapy reduces risk of heart disease in women after the menopause, but no trials of diet or weight reduction to prevent heart disease have been carried out with women.

Some studies suggest that certain types of cancer, particularly those of the gallbladder and the uterus, are more common in fat women. It is also said that breast cancer is linked to obesity. In fact, breast cancer is the major risk of death in pre-menopausal women, but it is more common in pre-menopausal women who are tall and thin. However, after the menopause breast cancer is slightly more common in women who are fat. There is currently little positive action women can take to avoid breast cancer.

The risk of several non-fatal disorders such as diabetes, gallstones, gout, varicose veins and osteoarthritis increases with being overweight, but the risks are much greater in the very fat than in the plump. Those men and women who have fat tummies and shoulders are more likely to develop diabetes, gout and heart disease than those who have fat bottoms and thin tops. So there is no doubt that keeping fat off the tummy and shoulders is good for your health. But fatness still has some advantages:

- Fatter women give birth to bigger babies. Current views suggest that big babies are less likely to suffer from heart disease and diabetes in later life.
- Fatter women are less likely to have problems breast-feeding.
- In the elderly, fatter people are less likely to suffer from hypothermia.
- Fatter people are less likely to suffer from fractures of vertebrae, hip, pelvis and femur because they are less likely to suffer from osteoporosis (brittle bones). Hip fracture is the greatest cause of disability in North American women and a major cause of death; it is 2.5 times less

likely to occur in fat women.

- Fat people are also more likely to survive a heart attack than thin people.
- Fat people are less susceptible to lung infections.

At the turn of the century, the romantic hero was a gaunt artist dying of tuberculosis (TB) in a garret. TB used to be the major cause of death in young adults until the Second World War, and was linked to poor diet and living conditions. TB is now re-emerging as a major public health problem in America. The spread of AIDS and the emergence of drug-resistant forms of TB are the major reasons. The World Health Organization is predicting a major world epidemic of tuberculosis. Fat people are less likely than thin people to develop fatal tuberculosis. A study of over 800,000 United States Navy recruits found that fat men were far more resistant to developing the disease. Other studies have confirmed that fatness is associated with a decreased risk from all infectious diseases. It perhaps confirms what has been known for years about children: that plump children are far more robust than those who are lean.

So, in conclusion, being underweight is a much more serious risk to health than being overweight. But being very overweight is harmful to health in that it increases the risk of a number of physical and medical disorders. Middle-aged men have to be particularly careful to avoid pot-bellies, because this increases their risk of dying prematurely from cardiovascular disease. Plumpness in young women has benefits in terms of increased survival and decreased morbidity (ill health).

Perils of Dieting

Until recently it was assumed that weight-loss is always beneficial. However, it now seems that the hazards associated with some of the treatments far outweigh the risks to health posed by obesity. There is little doubt that being seriously overweight increases the risk of dying prematurely and of suffering from a number of disabling conditions. However, it does not necessarily follow that weight-loss will reduce that increased risk – especially if it was the process of weight-gain that caused harm rather than the additional weight itself. It is a sad fact that most people who achieve weight-loss soon regain the weight. Several studies have found that people whose weights fluctuate markedly are at increased risk of heart disease compared with those who are overweight and whose weight does not fluctuate.

Weight fluctuations – known as yo-yo dieting – often involves rapid weight-loss. This is also bad for us. Here are examples of how this behaviour causes more harm than good, particularly in the severely obese:

- decreases in lean tissue (including heart muscle)
- loss of bone minerals
- attacks of gout or gallstones
- cardiac arrhythmias leading to sudden heart attacks
- hair-loss
- fibrosis and scarring of tissues
- refeeding hypertension (high blood pressure when returning to a normal diet)
- depression
- harmful side-effects of appetite-depressant drugs
- shortened life-span

A study of Japanese men in Hawaii found that those who were *lighter* in weight later in life than they had been at 25 were more likely to die prematurely. A massive study of one million adults by the American Cancer Society showed that people who claimed to have lost weight within the past five years were more likely to die from coronary heart disease than those whose weight was stable. In the Framingham study – another massive research project in the United States – people who lost 10 pounds after a heart attack (probably on the advice of their doctor) were twice as likely to die compared with those who had stable weights.

There are some examples where whole communities have been starved. The siege of Leningrad is a well-known case. Two years later when food again became available there was a rapid increase in the prevalence of high blood pressure and congestive heart failure. The starvation during the siege led to rapid weight-loss. This probably damaged body tissues impairing the body's system for controlling blood pressure. The dangers of fasting are highlighted by one hospital study of 200 fat men who were placed on a total fast, some for more than two months. After release from hospital the men regained all the weight they had lost. As they regained, 80 per cent developed diabetes and 25 per cent died – mainly of heart disease. Their death rate was thirteen times higher than would be expected of equally heavy men who had not dieted. This illustrates the hazards of crash dieting.

Invasion of the Body Snatchers

The medical profession has also been guilty of using drastic measures to treat obesity. They read like a list of medieval tortures. One example is surgery. This carries a high risk of complications. Many of these procedures became popular before they were properly evaluated in terms of safety and effectiveness:

- *Jaw wiring*. This is one drastic way to stop patients eating. However, many compulsive eaters liquidize their food and suck it through a straw.
- *Gastric balloon*. This involves placing an inflatable balloon

in the stomach so as to restrict the amount of food that can be eaten. Many experts aren't convinced about the effectiveness and safety of this procedure.

- *Banded gastroplasty.* Surgical reduction of size of the stomach. This operation carries a high risk of side-effects.
- *Ileal bypass.* Causes malabsorption of nutrients and gastrointestinal discomfort.
- *Liposuction.* Involves sucking the fat from underneath the skin. If it is not carried out properly, it can be extremely disfiguring. In some cases the fat grows back in lumps.

The Truth About Dieting

In this chapter we have looked at the reasons why people go on diets and the health risks of obesity. We have shown that preoccupation with body image is the major reason, not health. But it is quite natural for women to be fatter than men; indeed, it is essential for normal reproduction. So what are the real risks posed by fat to health?

- The hazards of obesity have been grossly exaggerated compared to other lifestyle factors such as smoking.
- To be very fat is undesirable because it increases the risk of several medical conditions that are not only life-threatening but reduce the quality of life.
- There are few hazards associated with plumpness and these are confined mainly to men with raised blood pressure, blood cholesterol and diabetes.
- As far as women are concerned, the health risks of being fat are minor and plumpness has advantages.
- The health risks of being very thin are much greater than those of being plump.
- Rapid weight-loss can be hazardous.
- Repeated weight-loss followed by weight-gain is even more hazardous.

Most doctors would agree that *maintaining* an acceptable weight is the best way to stay healthy. This means that **the diet industry does far more to threaten our health than to safeguard it**. When you see how our bodies gain and lose fat in the next chapter this becomes even clearer.

4   BODY FAT – HOW YOU GET IT, HOW YOU LOSE IT

In this chapter we look at the reasons why people put on weight and show you that fat is not a harmful substance but is essential for normal health. Depositing fat and losing fat are entirely natural processes which ensure the survival of the human race.

In Chapter 1 we highlighted the top ten myths used to sell diet books and diet products: for example, the idea that there was a special type of fat called cellulite which accumulated because of toxic substances in the diet or that certain combinations of foods would magically make body fat fade away. We then showed how we have become neurotic in our attitudes towards food and body shape. Some of us cannot resist temptation when over-exposed to food and put on weight; while others (those who usually have no need to lose weight) become excessive plate-watchers – they cease to enjoy food and put their health in danger by losing too much weight. We revealed research which shows that being underweight is a much more serious health problem than being slightly overweight. To regard plump women as unhealthy is completely wrong. *Fat* has become a dirty word – body fat is meant to be disgusting and dietary fat a killer. This is a travesty of fat's important role in maintaining good health. Let's first look at how fat fits, quite naturally, into our diets.

Food Facts

Food energy is most commonly measured in units called *kilocalories* (kilojoules are the metric equivalent and there are roughly 4 to each kilocalorie). Fat, protein, carbohydrate and alcohol are all used to power the body. These four elements give us our calories. When we eat or drink it is equivalent to recharging our batteries. Here is the amount of energy (kilocalories/gram) each of the building-blocks of an average diet supplies :

	Kilocalories per gram
Fat	9
Alcohol	7
Protein	4
Carbohydrate	3.75

Table 4.1

Their chemical energy is released when they are broken down in the body. A kilocalorie provided by fat is the same as that provided by carbohydrate. Some diet books try to pretend that the calories provided by fat are somehow different from those provided by the calories from carbohydrate or protein. That's as daft as saying that a pound of feathers is lighter than a pound of lead. Or that electricity generated by wind power is different from that generated by a coal-fired power station. Energy is energy whatever its form. What is true is that fat is the most concentrated source of calories.

Some foods contain a lot of water, such as lettuce or meat. Others, such as nuts and cereals, contain very little. Foods with a high water content are lower in food energy compared to those with a high fat content. As fat is a much more concentrated source of energy, foods high in fat are high in food energy. But the amount of nutrients provided by a food will, of course, depend upon how much is eaten. Table 4.2 shows the amounts of food energy, protein, carbohydrate, fat and water contained in a selection of common foods.

Food	Energy (kcal)	Protein (grams)	Carbohydrate (grams)	Fat (grams)	Water (grams)
Lettuce	14	0.80	1.70	0.50	95.00
Tomato	17	0.70	3.10	0.30	93.00
Apple	47	0.40	11.80	0.10	85.00
Potatoes	75	2.10	17.20	0.20	79.00
Cod, raw	76	17.40	0.00	0.70	82.00
Chicken meat	121	20.50	0.00	4.30	74.00
Lean beef	123	20.30	0.00	4.60	74.00
Egg	147	12.50	0.00	10.80	75.00
Wholemeal bread	215	9.30	41.60	2.50	38.00
Lentils, raw	297	24.30	48.80	1.90	11.00
Pasta, raw	324	13.40	66.20	2.50	10.00
Oatmeal, raw	375	11.20	66.00	9.20	8.00
Rice, raw	383	7.30	85.80	3.60	11.00
Sugar	394	0.00	105.00	0.00	0.00
Cheese	404	24.70	0.10	34.00	37.00
Soya beans	447	36.80	23.50	23.50	7.00
Peanuts	564	25.60	12.50	46.10	6.00
Butter	737	0.50	0.00	81.70	16.00
Cooking oil	894	0.00	0.00	99.30	0.00

Source: McCance and Widdowson's *The Composition of Foods*, 5th Edition

Table 4.2. Amounts of energy, protein, carbohydrate, fat and water per 100 grams of food

Some popular diet books refer to protein foods and carbohydrate foods, but this is misleading as most foods comprise mixtures of the nutrients (protein, fat, carbohydrates, vitamins and minerals). Only a few refined foods such as sugar and fat consist of merely one or two nutrients.

Our average daily diet consists of about forty different food items. Some of them are just variations of the same basic foodstuff, for example, milk and cheese (dairy) or bread and pasta (wheat). Human diets consist of mixtures of these basic foodstuffs:

- cereals (wheat, rice, corn, rye, millet, oats) and starchy foods (potatoes and other tubers)
- meat and fish
- milk products and eggs
- fruit and vegetables
- nuts and pulses (peas, beans and lentils)

Foods like sugar, fat and salt are used in cooking and food preparation to make foods taste nicer. Adding fat to food also greatly increases its food energy value. For example, spreading butter on bread doubles its calories. Decreasing fat intake can drastically lower energy intake. For example, a small glass of skimmed milk contains 40 kilocalories compared with 80 kilocalories in a glass of full cream milk.

Powering Up

The body needs energy to make muscles work and to maintain its different organs. The two main fuel sources are glucose and fat, although alcohol and protein can also be used. These fuels are burned up by reaction with the oxygen we breathe to provide the energy to drive the body. Carbon dioxide is generated in the process, which we exhale in our breath. The body uses fat as its main fuel most of the time. Some glucose is also used to generate energy, but much of it is stored in a form called glycogen in our liver and muscles. This can be used as an emergency fuel reserve. Glycogen is broken down to form glucose, which is then metabolized to provide energy during strenuous activity, when the normal supply of oxygen is insufficient for the body's needs.

What Exactly Is Body Fat?

Fat is nature's battery. It is a store of energy that can be used by the body when food intake is low or energy expenditure is high. When we eat more food energy than we use up we deposit what is unused as fat. Fat can be made in the body from carbohydrate or alcohol, or obtained directly from fat present in food. Fat is an extremely efficient way of storing energy as it is lighter than water and twice as concentrated in food energy as carbohydrate. The humps on the back of a camel consist of fat and they enable it to survive for long periods of time without food.

Storage fat is present in the body mainly as a fuel reserve, but it also protects and cushions delicate organs such as the kidneys. Storage fat is found mainly underneath the skin but also inside the abdominal cavity. Fat stored underneath the skin leads to the formation of dimples. The term *cellulite* was coined in the early 1970s by the French to describe the puckered appearance of fat on the tops of women's legs. There is nothing technical about cellulite; it's really just the French word for fat. Skin is attached to muscle by collagen fibrils in a mesh-like network, rather like a string vest. When fat is deposited it fills up the gaps leading to a dimply appearance. This dimply appearance becomes exaggerated as the overlying skin loses its elasticity with age and is exacerbated by excessive exposure to sunlight. The idea put forward in many diet books that 'toxins' have anything to do with the entirely natural process of fat deposition is absurd.

As we explained in the last chapter, body fat plays an important role in enabling reproduction in women. Reproduction cannot occur unless women have adequate stores of fat. This is possibly to ensure that the energy needed for pregnancy can be supplied. Most women put on about 2 stone in pregnancy. A large proportion of this is the baby, the placenta and amniotic fluid. The rest, about 4 kilograms (9 pounds), is body fat. Fat deposition in pregnancy is an entirely natural process and happens to all mammals. The fat acts as an energy store to help subsidize the energy cost of lactation. Each kilogram of body fat deposited during pregnancy can be cashed in during lactation to yield 7000 kilocalories, which is sufficient to support the cost in energy of producing 10 litres of milk (16 pints). That's enough to support a baby for about twenty-five days.

Infants have a large surface area relative to their weight and thus a greater surface area to lose heat from. Body fat plays an important role for them as an insulator in the newborn and helps reduce the loss of body heat. Premature infants do not lay down enough fat to keep them warm and so have to be kept in incubators. Newborn infants are also endowed with 'brown fat' which can oxidize to release energy as heat to help them keep warm. It is called brown fat because it contains many mitochondria (subcellular organelles that oxidize fat) which give it a brown colour. It is found mainly around the neck and between the shoulder-blades.

So fat acts as an important fuel reserve when energy demands are high. Many boys become slightly fat before the onset of puberty but then rapidly thin out. This is probably to ensure that they have enough energy for their adolescent growth-spurt.

How Do You Get Fat?

We get fat when we take in more food energy than we are using up. The rate at which we use up energy is determined by our body weight, age, sex and level of physical activity. Babies have very high rates of energy expenditure in relation to their body weight as they have a relatively large surface area from which to lose heat and they are growing rapidly. By the time we mature our surface area relative to weight decreases and we no longer have the energy cost of growth. We need a certain amount of energy to tick over. This resting energy expenditure is called *basal metabolic rate*. On top of this we have to add the energy cost of our level of physical activity. For example, a lumberjack has a very high level of activity compared with an office worker and will need almost twice as much food energy. Table 4.3 shows the energy expenditure of two different women who both run a home. One is sedentary and the other is active.

	Kilocalories/day	
	Active	Sedentary
Resting energy expenditure	1300	1300
Sleeping 8 hours	–	–
Housework 1 hour	100	100
Cycling 30 minutes	160	–
Walking 30 minutes	100	100
Swimming 30 minutes	190	–
Sitting	150	200
Total energy expenditure	2000	1700

Table 4.3

You can see that the woman who is more active uses up about 300 kilocalories more per day. If these two women ate the same amount of food energy at 2000 kilocalories per day, the woman who was sedentary would put on about 1 kilogram of fat in a month. There is good evidence that people who keep physically active are much more likely to maintain their weight.

As a nation we are getting fatter. But there is very little evidence to suggest that as a nation we are eating more. In fact most of the surveys find that energy intakes have decreased by about a third over the past forty years (Table 4.4.)

YEAR	Average daily kilocalorie intake
1945	2387
1950	2474
1955	2641
1960	2630
1965	2590
1970	2560
1975	2290
1980	2230
1985	2020
1990	1872

Source: MAFF

Table 4.4.

So our increasingly sedentary lifestyles must be one reason why we are putting on weight. The fatter people become, the more likely they are to lie about what they eat! A study published in the *New England Journal of Medicine* in 1993 found that very fat people under-estimated their energy intake and over-estimated their energy expenditure by up to 50 per cent.

It's important to realize that you don't get fat quickly and certainly not overnight. So don't think that because you have one blow-out of a meal all is lost. To put on 1 kilogram (2.2 pounds) of body fat you have to consume in excess of 10,000 kilocalories. That's equivalent to:

- 1¼ litres of oil or 3 half-pound packets of butter
  or
- 37 bars of chocolate (50 grams each)
  or
- 52 NutraSlim chocolate-coated meal replacement bars (50 grams each)
  or
- 40 Slender meal replacement bars (72 grams each)
  or
- 25 hamburgers
  or
- 75 cans of sugary drinks
  or
- 54 pints of beer
  or
- 50 cartons of Slim-Fast (300 ml each)
  or
- 35 packets of peanuts (50 grams each)
  or
- 158 rashers of streaky bacon
  or
- 135 chocolate digestive biscuits

or
- 27 pints of milk

or
- 113 eggs

or
- 5½ pounds of hard cheese

Adults often put on weight in cycles, usually a few weeks at a time. Typical times when people put on weight are:

- the Christmas period when there is more food and drink on offer and they are less physically active
- when away from home at a conference or on holiday, especially when the food is already paid for
- during pregnancy (this is quite natural)

There are many other reasons why people gain weight and become fatter but decreased physical activity is probably the most important factor:

- As we get older we become less active and expend less energy.
- There is an increased availability of high-energy food nowadays: snack trolleys at work, takeaway foods in shopping precincts and stations and automatic vending machines.
- In the late twentieth century cars, buses, lifts, escalators and other labour-saving devices (washing machines, vacuum cleaners, etc.) lead us to expend less energy doing day-to-day activities.
- Central heating and good clothing mean that we expend less energy keeping warm.
- Adults now sit in front of the television for an average of 25–30 hours a week.

Differences in Metabolism

Sudden unexpected weight-loss is generally associated with disease. There are many reasons why people lose weight when they are ill. Often it is because they don't feel well and their appetite is poor. Sometimes, however, it is the disease itself that is increasing the rate at which food energy is used. There are many diseases that lead to an increase in metabolic rate (the speed at which our bodies use up nutrients to provide us with energy) and cause weight-loss. Your body temperature rises when you have influenza for this very reason – your metabolism has increased.

Cancer is a disease that leads to severe weight-loss, but only part of the weight-loss can be explained by decreased appetite. There are also metabolic diseases that speed up our metabolic rate. President George Bush lost 12 pounds when he had Graves disease, a disease in which the thyroid gland is over-active and makes the body use much more energy than normal.

Various drugs are known to stimulate our metabolic rate but most of them have nasty side-effects. Smokers tend to be lighter in weight than non-smokers but they do not have a lower intake of food energy. It is the drug nicotine, present in cigarettes, which increases the metabolic rate. This is probably why smokers are lighter and why they put on 2–3 kilograms (4.4–6.6 pounds) when they give up smoking. Other drugs known to increase metabolic rate are ephidrine and bromocryptine. These drugs have unpleasant side-effects such as nausea and high blood pressure; while smoking, of course, causes cancer and heart disease.

Despite what is often said, most people who are fat don't have anything wrong with their glands. Nor do fat people have low metabolic rates. There is little evidence, either, for the idea that diet in childhood causes obesity in adulthood. The majority of teenagers are not overweight. Many of us start to put on weight in early adult life simply because our energy requirement falls as a result of decreased physical activity. Ideally we should maintain the weight we are in early adult life throughout life. Many men like to pretend that the paunches they acquire in middle age are solid muscle. This is rubbish. What they don't realize is that in men most of the fat is stored inside the belly.

There is no evidence that taking exercise boosts your metabolic rate as claimed in many popular diet books. However, the energy cost of regular physical activity probably can help prevent you getting fat. If you cycled for forty minutes, five days a week for forty weeks a year, that would use up an additional 60,000 kilocalories. If you stopped cycling and continued to eat as much you would put on about 6 kilograms (almost a stone) of body fat over a year.

How Much Weight Is It Possible to Lose?

In Chapter 1 we criticized many books and diet products for claiming excessive weight-losses. If you cut down your energy intake by 1000 kilocalories per day for a week, you will lose 1 kilogram (2.2 pounds) in body weight. An average man needs about 2300 kilocalories a day. If he fasted and drank only water, he would lose 2.3 kilograms (5.6 pounds) of body fat in a week. Fasting, besides being dangerous, is not recommended for weight-loss because it leads to a loss of lean tissue like muscle. This gradually winds down your metabolic rate. As a result, when you start eating normally again your body needs fewer calories, so you put on weight more easily. It can also increase the risk of developing high blood pressure (commonly called *refeeding hypertension*).

Fashionable meal replacements, which are typically sachets of powder or biscuits, claim rapid weight-loss (for example, up to 4 pounds a week is claimed by one leading

Rate of weight loss in men and women on 1000 kilocalories/day diet

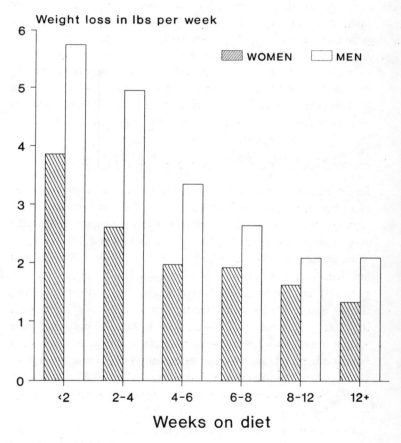

Sample size 854

Figure 4.1

brand). As soon as people stop using them most people put the weight back on again. It is better to be continually plump than to allow your weight to yo-yo.

Experts are generally agreed that if you need to lose weight it is best to do it gently. Effective weight-reducing diets provide between 1000 and 1600 kilocalories a day depending upon sex, weight and age. When you cut your energy intake down your body uses the energy stored in your body fat. But it still needs the other nutrients like protein, vitamins and minerals to keep you healthy. If the diet contains inadequate protein, then muscle tissue will be broken down. It is quite possible to get all the nutrients you need on a 1000-kilocalorie-a-day diet but it does need careful planning. For weight reduction to be effective and maintained, dietary advice also needs to be accompanied by a change of behaviour towards food and eating.

We looked at the records of a commercial slimming club which gave dietary advice and behavioural-modification therapy. We studied the rate at which several hundred people lost weight on a sensible 1000–1200-kilocalorie-a-day diet. On average men lost 1.3 kilograms per week (2.9 pounds) and women 0.8 kilograms per week (1.8 pounds). The rate of weight-loss was greatest in the first three weeks of the diet and then tailed off (Figure 4.1).

There are several reasons why this happens. In the first week much of the weight-loss is water not fat. After that most of the weight-loss is fat. As weight is lost so the body adapts to requiring less food energy and the rate of weight-loss falls. On a diet such as this it takes a man about three to four months to lose 2 stone and a woman four to five months. We found the rates of weight-loss were almost exactly as we predicted. Less dramatic reductions in energy intake (300–400 kilocalories a day) still lead to considerable weight-loss in the long term. Indeed, this is what happens when people give up dieting and bingeing and begin to eat sensibly.

Exercise

Many people are under the illusion that taking more regular exercise will make you lose lots of weight. While there are many good reasons for taking regular exercise, as we pointed out earlier, it only makes a small contribution to weight-loss. To lose 1 kilogram (2.2 pounds) of body fat you would have to expend an additional 7000 kilocalories. Moderate exercise, such as cycling for forty minutes a day, uses up only 300 kilocalories. So to lose 1 kilogram of body fat you would have to cycle for about sixteen hours – or at least forty minutes a day for twenty-three days. On the other hand, decreasing your food energy intake by 1000 kilocalories a day would lead to a loss of 1 kilogram in a week.

It is possible to increase the amount of fat lost slightly by taking more physical exercise. If you take light exercise three times a week, say, for forty to forty-five minutes, this will make you lose about 100 grams (4 ounces). However, there is no need to become a fitness freak to lose weight. Exercise can improve muscle tone but it can't make you lose fat from selected areas like the hips and thighs. You don't have to do all those silly exercises with your bum in the air or your legs behind your ears!

Many people who are fat or overweight regard gyms with their racks and bars as medieval torture chambers. Sport isn't necessarily the best way to increase your physical activity. Most heart specialists agree that the best exercise is the mild type – just enough to increase your pulse rate but not so severe that you can't talk because of lack of breath. It is far better to take mild exercise regularly than heavy exercise occasionally. If you are very overweight, taking up squash is not a good idea. Squash is very intense exercise and can precipitate a stroke or heart attack. One doctor remarked that the only exercise he had taken recently was being pallbearer at the funerals of his squash-playing friends. Light exercise such as cycling, walking and swimming is far better. Jogging is not such a good idea if you are very overweight as it puts a strain on your joints. Swimming is probably the best exercise for fat people because the fat keeps you warm and helps you float. It is the only form of exercise where fatness can be an advantage. Just think of seals and walruses!

The Importance of Fat in the Diet

Most diet books suggest that fat is an undesirable component of the diet. This is completely wrong. Fat makes food palatable, it is a useful source of energy (especially when demands are high), it is essential for the provision and absorption of the fat-soluble vitamins and has an indispensable role in providing essential fatty acids.

Avoiding fat in the diet does not guarantee that you will lose weight, because alcohol and carbohydrate-rich foods such as bread, rice, sugar and potatoes can also be converted into fat in the body. **Feeding children under the age of 5 on low-fat diets is particularly dangerous as this restricts their energy intake and can stunt their growth**.

Recommendations have been made by governments throughout the world to decrease the intake of saturated fatty acids in order to reduce the risk of heart disease. It is generally accepted that men should cut down on their intake of fats rich in saturated fatty acids (those which are solid at room temperature – lard, solid vegetable fat, meat fat) because they increase blood-cholesterol levels. These recommendations were based on studies in men, not in women. Prior to the menopause heart disease is rare in women and blood-cholesterol levels are low. We carried out a study with healthy women and asked them to cut down on their total fat intake, particularly the saturated type. Although they succeeded in cutting down on fat quite markedly, it had no influence on their blood-cholesterol levels. What's good for the gander may not be so good for the goose. And yet the diet trade aims its products and books much more at women than at men, all the while peddling specious fears about dietary fat.

The fat in butter, milk and cheese is a good source of vitamin A, vegetable oils are the richest source of vitamin E, oil-rich fish are the best dietary source of vitamin D. Fat is also needed to enable the absorption of these fat-soluble vitamins – beta-carotene (the form of vitamin A found in plant foods) is poorly absorbed on low-fat diets. We need about 30 grams of fat a day to absorb the vitamins properly. In parts of the world where low-fat diets are eaten, vitamin A deficiency is common. One of the authors, in a letter to *The Lancet* in 1990, pointed out that vitamin A levels are inadequate in many young women because they are switching to low-fat dairy products and avoiding foods such as liver. Although low-fat spreads are fortified with vitamin A and D, other low-fat dairy products are often devoid of the vitamins. A study published in July 1993 in the *New England Journal of Medicine* found that women with low intakes of vitamin A were at increased risk of breast cancer. Other studies published in the same journal, also in 1993, found that vitamin E may offer protection from heart disease and that vitamin D may help prevent osteoporosis. So all our diets need fat in them, not least to enable us to get the benefit of several key vitamins.

Fat also has a vital role in supplying certain polyunsaturated fatty acids which the body cannot make and needs for its normal metabolism. These are called the *essential fatty acids* and they are found in foods like nuts, oilseeds (and therefore vegetable oils such as sunflower oil) and oil-rich fish (mackerel, herring, sardines, salmon). These foods have been actually prohibited in some popular low-fat diets! The essential fatty acids are needed for making up the membranes in cells and for producing hormone-like substances in the body called prostaglandins and leukotrienes. Ideally we need about 15 grams a day of these polyunsaturated fatty acids and certainly not less than 4 grams. Studies have found that people who eat nuts and oil-rich fish regularly are less likely to suffer heart disease. A study carried out by Dr Michael Burr of the Medical Research Council found that giving advice to eat oil-rich fish twice a week to men who had previously suffered a heart attack reduced their risk of dying in the subsequent two years by 29 per cent. Giving them advice to cut down on fat had no benefit.

Conclusion

In this chapter we have explained why you get fat and how you lose it. We have explained that fat is not a harmful or toxic substance that occurs in the body. Fat is nature's battery. It is perfectly normal to lay down fat and to mobilize it when you need it. People gain weight because their intake is not balanced by their energy expenditure. Conversely, weight is lost when energy expenditure exceeds energy intake. The rate of both weight-gain and weight-loss is predictable. Fat is not only a desirable but also an essential element in the diet and provides several nutrients that keep us healthy. So great is the level of misinformation from diet quacks and profiteers that *fat* has become a dirty word. Even worse, its very mention can often provoke feelings of guilt and self-revulsion. Is it any wonder that the incidence of eating disorders is increasing so rapidly?

5 EATING DISORDERS

Until recently anorexia was the disorder which received all the publicity. But, in fact, bulimia is now much more common, and millions suffer from milder eating disorders such as bingeing or other unhealthy eating patterns caused by dieting. This chapter looks at the range of eating disorders and how they can be cured.

We tend to think of eating disorders as extreme conditions which only afflict other people. But answer these questions:

- Do you frequently go on diets?
- How often do you tell other people: 'I mustn't, I'm on a diet'?
- Do you often count calories?
- Does your weight fluctuate regularly – losing a stone on a diet, then putting it on again and so on?
- Do you ever have eating binges – like consuming five Mars bars at one sitting?
- Do you often prepare one meal for family or friends and a totally different one for yourself?
- Do you often eat separately and secretly from the rest of your family or friends?
- Have you ever turned down an invitation because you couldn't face dealing with the food?
- Do you find you are obsessed with food all day long?
- Do you ever feel nervous, anxious or guilty about what you eat?

Many people reading this book will have answered Yes to some or all of those questions. And, while we are not suggesting that they need hospital treatment, it is a fact that anyone 'on a diet' is losing touch with their body's natural instinct for food.

This is indeed a form of eating disorder, if a mild one. We have already written about how the cycle of dieting and bingeing (putting on weight, dieting again and so on) is very bad for our bodies. But it is also bad for our minds. We learn to regard food as forbidden fruit, to feel guilty and to deny our natural feelings of hunger. Then, in compensation, we binge and eat huge amounts of food that bear no relation to our hunger or our body's need. This is not normal and may result from some unhappiness in our lives. But it is also a disorder that the diet industry is responsible for aiding and abetting. There is another way, and in the final chapter we take you through it. It is designed to help those of us who are stuck in the cycle of despair, yo-yoing between famine diets on the one hand and binge eating on the other.

If you feel you cannot break out of this cycle of despair on your own there is now help. Eating Disorder Units in National Health hospitals only deal with extreme eating disorders such as bulimia and anorexia. But others have now recognized that the diet mania and the distorted eating patterns that go with it are a disorder and that they can dominate their victims' lives in a very extreme way. Here are some of the organizations you can contact for help:

Dietbreakers Send a stamped addressed envelope to Diet-breakers, Church Cottage, Barford St Michael, Oxon OX15 0YA. Founded in 1992 by Mary Evans Young, who was shocked by the suicide of a 15-year-old who was bullied for being size 14. Apart from campaigning on diet issues she offers courses called 'Do You Really Need to Diet?' and 'You Count – Calories Don't'. The courses encourage self-confidence and challenge the assumption that fat is bad and thin is good.

Maisner Centre for Eating Disorders, Box 464, Hove, East Sussex, BN3 2BN (0273 329334). Paulette Maisner was herself a bulimic. Dieting makes you fat and following diets makes you ill, she says. She treats compulsive eaters as well as bulimics. She helps people to increase their self-esteem and forget about their weight. They use daily plans to help establish normal eating patterns.

Overeaters Anonymous, PO Box 19, Stratford, Manchester M32 9EB. Founded in the United States in 1960 and run along the same lines as Alcoholics Anonymous. There are now around a hundred self-funding groups in Britain. Members meet regularly to discuss their problems and how to deal with them. They look at the emotional and psychological problems that relate to eating disorders. Diets, they say, can be the *cause* of over-eating.

Weigh Ahead, 2 The Crescent, Busby, Glasgow G76 8HT (041-644 1444). Cherie Martin, Weigh Ahead's founder, suffered personally from alternate dieting and bingeing for many years. At Weigh Ahead in Glasgow she runs courses at which she helps people achieve permanent weight control. Among the key steps are never dieting again, finding out why you over-eat and learning how to manage stress.

The people who attend these organizations (and they are by no means only women) invariably discover that they only lose weight permanently *after* they give up dieting and return to normal eating. That is something we explore in the next chapter.

How Ill Can You Get?

It may be that, like the majority of people, you have never suffered from what doctors, up to now, have called an eating disorder – bulimia or anorexia. But a significant minority do now suffer from these more extreme diseases. Read the words of actual sufferers below and you will begin to understand the inner torment that it involves:

'I made sure my work was excellent – the desire for perfection is part of the anorectic condition. Provided your work was good, those in charge couldn't approach you, even if they were a bit suspicious. I could sit vomiting at one end and having diarrhoea at the other, thinking I was really in control.'

'You really get high on being anorectic. In a way you feel you have achieved something. It becomes a challenge.'

'I had narrowed my life to this strict schedule. Food was the only thing I could control. I felt I had control over my life.'

'I wasn't going home much because of all the friction, so I wasn't eating properly. And all the time I was getting thinner and thinner. What I liked about that was that it was something I could do on my own. I could live in my own little world and be in control without having to get approval or permission . . . Yet at the same time I was completely obsessed by food. I would cook for other people, make wonderful meals. I'd spend hours in supermarkets looking at the stuff, studying the calories, but I wouldn't eat any of it.'

'When I look in the mirror I agree that I'm thin, but I don't think I'd ever be comfortable with a physical appearance of health and radiating blissful contentment when I don't feel like that inside . . . What you see is how I feel inside.'

'My life was in limbo and I became very frightened of death. I used to curl up in bed. I was going into a kind of emptiness and my body was going into an emptiness as well because it was shrinking. But I felt that was beautiful.'

'I used to get my mum to weigh my food for me in minute portions. I hated the feeling of it in my stomach. It all started when a colleague at work called me "pleasantly plump". From then on I wanted to be thin. I got so bony people were shocked. But when they said, "God, you look thin," I was flattered not worried. I was out of control of my eating habits but I loved to be thin.'

'Every minute you're awake the only thing you think about is food. You can't sleep for more than a couple of hours because of your hunger. It's the only thing in your life.'

'I kept looking in the mirror and all I could see were big bulges. I was getting really good at disguising the fact that I wasn't eating and I didn't want people to see me eating. I didn't want it to be seen as if I had given in. I'd feel guilty then, as if I'd broken the vow . . .'

'I was completely trapped by food. You think about it all the time, and when you aren't thinking about it you are eating enormous quantities of it. Part of the cause was boredom, which is a big factor for most bulimics. I also felt guilty when I ate.'

'Unless you have experienced an eating disorder it is difficult to know what it is all about. The vomiting, over-eating, starvation and purging are just the symptoms of underlying emotional problems. What you have to realize is that those feelings cannot be solved, they are part of life that you cannot escape – the sufferer has to realize that in order to start on the path to recovery.'

Amongst those sufferers we have quoted are the teenage girl who was 5 foot 6 inches but only 5 stone and whose daily diet was two apples and six cans of Diet Coke; and the man who was 6 feet tall, weighed only 7 stone and who ate one bowl of muesli a day which he often threw up. If any of the feelings towards food expressed here mirror you own, then you need help. And you can get help, as one of the sufferers we quoted is quick to point out: *'They think they can't recover, which is wrong. They are desperate.'*

There are two conditions named above – anorexia and bulimia. But it would be a mistake to regard them as two slightly different manifestations of the same problem. Dr Janet Treasure is Senior Lecturer in Eating Disorders at the Maudsley Hospital in London. She says that bulimia is massively on the increase and is ten times more common than anorexia. She points to two studies that have now proved bulimia is an illness caused by dieting. Anorexia, on the other hand, is much rarer and its causes are more difficult to tie down. So what is bulimia?

Bulimia Nervosa

Bulimia nervosa means 'eating like an ox through nervous-ness'. Anorectics often become bulimics. Bulimia is chiefly associated with:

- bingeing on large amounts of food, particularly 'forbid-den' foods such as biscuits, cakes, chocolate, nuts and crisps
- subsequent remorse
- doing anything to combat the excess calories from the bingeing sessions including starvation, self-induced vomiting, compulsive exercise and excessive use of laxa-tives (as many as a hundred a day)
- acute sensitivity to weight-change and body shape

Some long-term bulimics do not need to put two fingers down their throat to vomit – they can vomit at will. Unlike anorectics, sufferers do not tend to be underweight. They control their body weight by compulsive over-eating and then purging. Some of the symptoms are similar to anorexia but there are specific health problems:

- constant vomiting causes mineral deficiencies in the body, particularly potassium and sodium
- stomach acid passing through the mouth dissolves tooth enamel and causes advanced tooth decay
- puffy face caused by swollen salivary glands
- irregular heartbeats
- muscle weakness
- kidney damage
- stomach rupture
- dehydration
- epileptic fits
- laxative abuse can lead to persistent stomach pains and long-term constipation

Bulimia has been estimated to affect as many as 100,000 women aged between 15 and 45. Bulimics tend to be older than anorectics – typically women in their early to middle twenties who were overweight as children. It is particularly common amongst career women and it is on the increase. Male bulimia is also rising.

How to Spot Bulimia

Bulimia is more difficult to spot than anorexia because it is not usually associated with extreme weight-loss. In fact bulimics will go to great lengths to conceal their problem. The major tell-tale signs are:

- tooth decay
- puffy face
- large fluctuations in body weight

- vomiting marks on the knuckles from when the hand is raised to the mouth

How to Get Help

Often anorectics and bulimics will not admit they have a problem. If they do admit it, then just as often they don't want to be helped. If you are a parent and you fear your teenage child has an eating disorder, immediate confrontation may not be the right approach. It can lead to a sudden emotional upheaval and may be too painful an experience. It is best to get advice first.

So, if you are bulimic and you are prepared to do something about it or if you want advice on how to help someone else, this is where to go.

Your first port of call must be your GP; most doctors are now familiar with this growing problem and can approach it sympathetically. GPs worth their salt should spot the symptoms of bulimia anyway.

The GP can refer the sufferer or a parent to a psychiatrist or straight to hospital if the condition is serious. Not all NHS hospitals are very well equipped to deal with eating disorders but, if you can afford it, some private hospitals are now specializing in this area.

In the absence of a local hospital or psychiatrist known to have experience of treating eating disorders there will always be a community dietician or psychiatric nurse who could help. School doctors are also getting better at dealing with these problems.

If you feel that your GP is not really helping and there is not adequate support locally, then contact one of the following:

The Eating Disorders Association, Sackville Place, 44 Magdalen Street, Norwich, Norfolk NR3 1JE. Helpline Tel. 0603 621414. Youth Helpline (for under-18s) Tel. 0603 765050.

Anorexia & Bulimia Nervosa Association, Annexe C, Tottenham Town Hall, Town Hall Approach Road, London N15 4RX. Tel. 081-885 3936.

The Priory Centre, 11 Priory Road, High Wycombe, Bucks HP13 6SL. Tel. 0494 523440. It has a helpline and can counsel sufferers and their families. They also have thirty-five local self-help groups in Britain.

Most areas also have 'Wellwoman' clinics whose number can be found in the telephone book. To find reputable counselling in your area you can contact:

The British Association for Counselling, 37a Sheep Street, Rugby, Warwickshire CV21 3BX.

Finally a very good self-help book is available: *Self-Help in Bulimics* by Dr H. Lacey. It costs £5 from: Department of Mental Health Sciences, St George's Hospital Medical School, Tooting, London SW17.

Anorexia Nervosa

Anorexia nervosa actually means 'loss of appetite through nervousness', although sufferers usually have a normal appetite which they have suppressed. Anorexia is chiefly associated with:

- a self-induced starvation weight-loss
- a strong desire to be thinner and thinner
- an obsessive fear of weight-gain
- feeling fat even when emaciated

The medical cost of starvation is unpleasant and can be fatal. Symptoms may include:

- broken sleep
- feeling cold all the time
- loss of periods
- growth of facial hair
- sterility
- low blood pressure
- flatulence
- diarrhoea
- a dysfunctioning immune system
- vitamin and mineral deficiencies leading to anaemia and osteoporosis
- heart problems

Anorexia can be fatal: sufferers have starved to death, committed suicide or died from heart disease later on in life.

What Causes Anorexia?

As with most psychological problems there is a host of theories. Anorexia is particularly prevalent amongst teenage girls. It is entirely normal for them to put on weight around their hips and thighs after puberty. But everywhere they look – teenage magazines, street hoardings, television advertisements – they see incredibly thin women. 'Thin' is beautiful and only 'slim' is socially acceptable. So they reject what is, in fact, their perfectly natural body shape and start dieting. Some psychologists see anorexia as a way in which teenagers reject their change in body shape; in other words, they are frightened of growing up. Others regard anorexia as a way in which teenagers can exercise some control over their life in a world which seems completely out of their control.

Teenagers who diet should only do so under medical supervision. They should not be allowed into slimming clubs. And anyone who goes into a slimming club should NEVER take their children with them. A survey in London showed that at any one time one in three 15-year-old schoolgirls claimed to be dieting. *It has been estimated that the risk of a dieter developing an eating disorder is around eight times higher than for a non-dieter.*

Anorexia can be the way in which some other problem or anxiety manifests itself. The sufferer might be depressed, guilty, obsessional, lonely or upset at some disruption in their family or love life. And those who have a professional interest in food, such as caterers and dietitians, are more likely to suffer from anorexia. There are also high rates of anorexia amongst dancers and models, for whom it is essential to be slim. Anorexia may be less common than bulimia, but it has been estimated that 1 per cent of schoolgirls suffer from anorexia and as many as 3 per cent experience some of the symptoms. Anorexia can also afflict people right up to their forties. As we have seen, it can also affect men but it is ten times more likely in women.

How to Spot Anorexia

There are a number of clues – some are physical symptoms and others are behavioural:

- weight-loss
- powerful breath odour
- female facial hair
- claiming to be fat when actually thin
- reduction in food intake coupled with . . .
- greater interest in food and calories
- cooking for others but not eating personally
- eating very small amounts
- anxiety and arguments about over-eating when tiny amounts are involved (e.g. three peas rather than four)

- hiding uneaten food
- arguments at meal-times

The same organizations quoted above as helping bulimics will also help people with anorexia. There is also a self-help book, *Anorexia and the Wish to Change* by Dr A. Crisp. This is also available, for £5, from St George's Hospital in Tooting.

How Eating Disorders Are Treated

As we have pointed out, eating disorders are often caused by other problems in the sufferer's life. So diverse are these that it is not possible to comment on them except to say that eating disorders will return if such underlying problems are not identified and tackled. But here we are going to describe how anorexia and bulimia are physically treated.

Anorectics and bulimics are fascinated and obsessed by food. So they quite commonly adopt faddy, even bizarre, food regimes. Returning to sensible balanced eating has to be the primary objective. Where food is concerned sufferers should:

- eat several times a day
- stop taking laxatives
- increase fluid intake but beware of drinking too much coffee, tea or Coke because they are diuretics and can cause dehydration
- make sure foods eaten include a reasonable amount of carbohydrates such as bread, potatoes, pasta and rice
- in the case of those who have become vegetarian to avoid calories, slowly return to fish and meat or at least ensure that pasta and dairy products are consumed regularly

Other elements of treatment include:

- establishing a target weight with the GP or other counsellor
- aiming for a weight-gain of about 1 pound a week

- weekly weigh-ins to monitor the gain
- keeping of a diary to record food intake and any vomiting or bingeing (this brings back a feeling of control)

To help regularize eating habits doctors will often recommend a range of eating plans. Three are recommended in *Anorexia and the Wish to Change* by Dr Crisp:

- Plan A is 1000-1100 calories a day – a short-term regime that will not overstress the bodies of the very underweight
- Plan B is 1500-1600 calories a day – designed for stabilizing weight
- Plan C is 2000-2100 calories for weight-gain

So a sufferer might start on Plan A to get going, go on to Plan C for weight-gain and finally adopt Plan B to ensure a sensible consistent approach to eating. To that end they may have to eat even when they don't feel hungry. Crucially, Dr Crisp's plan offers a pathway to follow.

Curing eating disorders is, above all, a battle for the hearts and minds of sufferers. Key pieces of advice for them are:

- make any changes, like eating more and putting on weight, very gradually
- when you start to eat more don't be afraid of suddenly becoming fat – it takes far longer to put on weight than it does to lose it
- come to terms with what 'normal' weight is for someone of your height (see the Height/Weight Chart on p.95)
- remember that being considerably underweight is far, far more dangerous to your health than being mildly plump

Conclusion

What a happy world the diet industry has created. Diet books and products may not always be the original cause of eating disorders – that often comes from a deep-seated unhappiness – but the diet racketeers encourage eating disorders, cause misery and then, in an unvirtuous circle, profit from that misery. Dr Janet Treasure says that the diet industry is a capitalist dream: it churns out products that don't work. But the more they fail, the more people want them and so it goes on.

Much better public education is needed to counter diet propaganda and prevent eating disorders occurring at all. Schools are an obvious place to start, but the job has to be done very carefully so that, by explaining eating disorders, we are not providing a hook on which adolescents can hang their neuroses.

In this chapter we have shown how extreme eating disorders can become. But now we should return to the thought that *anyone* who goes in for prolonged dieting is suffering from an eating disorder of sorts. How can we all shake the habit and realize that we don't have to diet?

6 YOU DON'T HAVE TO DIET!

Nothing but sorrow and ill health come from constant dieting. To go on crash weight-loss programmes by restricting your intake of calories is unnatural and potentially dangerous. In this chapter, we are not offering any simplistic ten-point plan or short-term regime. Our aim is to help you to get back to a normal pattern of eating long-term and, most of all, to enjoy your food. Much of what we have to say is common sense – the most powerful antidote there is to the diet industry.

A 'balanced diet' was the phrase used by nutritionists to describe a mixture of foods that prevented nutritional deficiencies and promoted health. Nowadays the word *diet* has been hijacked by the weight-loss industry to sell books that can cause malnutrition and products that can seriously damage our health. Most bestselling diet books encourage bizarre eating patterns and thus encourage the consumption of unbalanced diets in order to attain body shapes unachievable by the majority. These self-appointed diet gurus with their misguided beliefs and homespun philosophy have attracted millions of acolytes who sacrifice their health for the glittering prize of slenderness. It is not the type of food we eat that is to blame but our attitude towards it. We are often ignorant about selecting a 'balanced diet', and many of us are simply physically inactive. It is a sad state of affairs that we now regard being unhealthily slim as evidence of well-being. The racketeers have ensnared many – particularly women – in the diet trap. They have undermined their confidence in food and their natural ability to regulate weight. But the failure of the dieting industry is plain to see from the ever-increasing proportion of people who are becoming obese. If current trends continue, one-quarter of the adult population will be obese by the year 2000. *Dieting is the problem, not the solution.*

Drastic remedies are rarely the solution to simple problems. You cannot cure yourself of eating too much by eating too little. Excessive prohibition and deprivation actually lead to over-compensation – in other words, yo-yo diets. Depriving yourself of foods you enjoy and living on a monotonous, tasteless diet of cottage cheese, crispbread, lettuce and skimmed milk is no fun whatsoever. It is only natural that people compensate by bingeing on tasty foods which are usually high in calories and fat. But, in fact, a little of what you fancy genuinely does you good, both emotionally and nutritionally. And only small changes in eating habits and physical activity are usually necessary to establish and maintain a healthy weight. In short, you don't have to diet.

All Shapes and Sizes

In this book, we have concentrated on emphasizing the hazards of being underweight, but we should equally avoid being seriously overweight. Ideally we should maintain the body weight of our early adulthood throughout life. There is no doubt that people who do this are generally healthier and age more gently. Preventing significant weight-gain in middle age is a desirable goal because it improves fitness and quality of life as well as preventing fatal illnesses.

We need to accept that we come in all shapes and sizes. There is nothing wrong with being plump, it is extreme slenderness that is unnatural and unhealthy. You must come to terms with the shape nature has endowed you with. If you are plump and happy then there is no need to bother about losing weight. If you are worried about your appearance, just make sure you buy clothes that fit comfortably – don't set yourself unrealistic goals. Don't blame your shape for other things you are unhappy about in your life.

Define them and face them – don't take it out on your body. On the other hand, if you are severely overweight (Body Mass Index over 30, see page 98) then you need to change your attitude towards food and not kid yourself that there are any short-term miracle cures.

The Balancing Act

It is time we reclaimed the word *diet* from the 'diet' industry. What it really should mean is a balanced diet. Diet in the broader (and real) sense of the word is important to maintain health. We need a balanced diet to provide all the nutrients the body requires as well as to prevent diet-related diseases such as heart disease, dental caries, cancer and bowel disease.

- We need to eat a variety of foods (meat, fish, dairy products, cereals, fruit and vegetables) to get all the nutrients we require.
- Avoiding heart disease involves eating less saturated fat of the type found in meat, dairy fat and solid vegetable fats and eating more oil-rich fish, and using liquid vegetable oils (such as sunflower oil) for cooking.
- Starchy foods and fruit and vegetables are believed to help protect against cancer and bowel disease.
- Avoiding the frequent consumption of sugary foods between meals helps prevents tooth decay.

Besides consuming a variety of foods we need to consider the relative proportions of foods we eat. We also talked about the food pyramid (see p.66) which puts emphasis on eating more starchy foods such as pasta, bread and rice, and fruit and vegetables. Most people have a limited repertoire of meals. They typically have the same thing for breakfast almost every day and on average they have seven to eight different types of main meal. So, if you want to change what you eat, all you have to do is dream up some different meals. We all have our likes and dislikes, and we are not going to dictate to you what you *must* eat. That's the preserve of the diet racketeers. It's up to you to make the choice, but make it a sensible one.

Appetite for Change

If you do put on weight easily, you need to change those food habits that caused the problem in the first place. Controlling your weight means:

- knowing which foods are most fattening
- knowing how to control portion size
- having a regular pattern of eating
- changing your attitude towards food

In most cases only small changes in your eating habits are necessary. Maintaining weight is about having control over what you eat. It is a continuous task. It is easier for some people than for others. For example, some people gain weight more easily than others. But it also depends upon a number of factors that you can influence:

- your attitude towards food – avoiding both over- and under-eating
- how physically active you are
- your lifestyle in general
- your frame of mind

Most people will always need to keep an eye on their weight. This doesn't mean you must never over-indulge in a favourite food. One fear that many people have is that they will rapidly put on weight if they eat a certain food, the fear that they will go to bed thin and wake up the next morning fat. We'd like to reassure you that the pounds simply don't reappear overnight like toadstools after rain. They sneak on a pinch at a time. This fear of a rapid weight-gain is what drives many people towards disorderly eating. It is a good idea to record your weight fortnightly. There is no point weighing yourself any more frequently as you won't see any change over such a short period of time.

Food Facts

Learning to control your weight means understanding how food provides energy. You don't have to become neurotic counting calories but you do need to have a feel for the calorific value of foods. It is best to think of food portions in terms of calorie equivalents. Table 6.1 shows the portions of food that provide the same number of calories. It will help you begin to judge the relative calorific value of different foods.

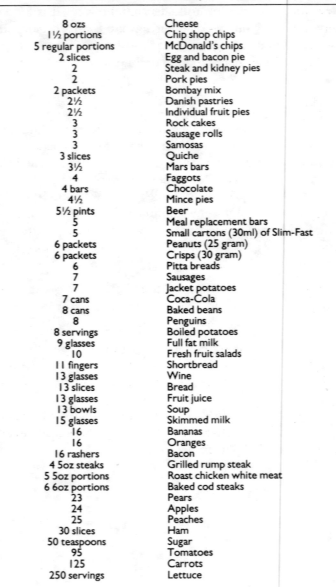

8 ozs	Cheese
1½ portions	Chip shop chips
5 regular portions	McDonald's chips
2 slices	Egg and bacon pie
2	Steak and kidney pies
2	Pork pies
2 packets	Bombay mix
2½	Danish pastries
2½	Individual fruit pies
3	Rock cakes
3	Sausage rolls
3	Samosas
3 slices	Quiche
3½	Mars bars
4	Faggots
4 bars	Chocolate
4½	Mince pies
5½ pints	Beer
5	Meal replacement bars
5	Small cartons (30ml) of Slim-Fast
6 packets	Peanuts (25 gram)
6 packets	Crisps (30 gram)
6	Pitta breads
7	Sausages
7	Jacket potatoes
7 cans	Coca-Cola
8 cans	Baked beans
8	Penguins
8 servings	Boiled potatoes
9 glasses	Full fat milk
10	Fresh fruit salads
11 fingers	Shortbread
13 glasses	Wine
13 slices	Bread
13 glasses	Fruit juice
13 bowls	Soup
15 glasses	Skimmed milk
16	Bananas
16	Oranges
16 rashers	Bacon
4 5oz steaks	Grilled rump steak
5 5oz portions	Roast chicken white meat
6 6oz portions	Baked cod steaks
23	Pears
24	Apples
25	Peaches
30 slices	Ham
50 teaspoons	Sugar
95	Tomatoes
125	Carrots
250 servings	Lettuce

Number of Portions of Food that provide 1000 Calories

Table 6.1

You should be able to see from this list that cheese, biscuits, pastry and fatty meat products contain lots of calories. Whereas lean meat, fish, bread and cereals contain far fewer, and fruit and vegetables contain hardly any.

We have found that men and women who maintain their weight on average consume 2300 and 1800 kilocalories per day respectively. Typically this is supplied as a main meal providing 800–1000 kilocalories and two smaller meals of 300–500 kilocalories each with snacks making up the balance. Typically the weight of food consumed is about 1 kilogram per day so the amount of food provided per 100 grams of diet is on average 180–200 kilocalories.

Many foods now have the energy value printed on the label in the box of nutritional information. Usually it is presented as kilocalories per 100 gram. As a rule of thumb food portions or serving can be divided up into those that are low, medium and high:

Low-calorie foods: less than 100 kilocalories per 100 grams
Medium-calorie foods: 100–250 kilocalories per 100 grams
High-calorie foods: More than 250 kilocalories per 100 grams

Some labels also give the number of kilocalories per portion. This is particularly useful if you are trying to judge ready-prepared meals. If you get into the habit of always reading the nutritional label on food products, and always judging whether it's low, medium or high calorie, then you will be well on the way to changing your eating habits for ever. Look at the examples in Table 6.2 (overleaf):

Food	kilocalories per 100g	kilocalories per portion
Low-calorie foods		
1 apple	35	42
1 banana	47	63
1 orange	26	64
Medium-calorie foods		
2 slices of ham	120	66
1 boiled egg	147	88
1 scoop of ice-cream	195	146
1 baked potato	105	147
2 slices of bread	219	153
1 serving of pasta	113	170
1 serving of rice	123	203
1 lean steak	167	260
1 slice of pizza	235	376
High-calorie foods		
1 portion of butter/margarine	737	59
1 small packet of crisps	533	166
1 Mars bar	441	287
1 50g packet of peanuts	572	286
2 Carnation Slender bars	350	250
1 Slim-Fast Fruit and Nut crunch bar	385	108
1 NutraSlim milk chocolate-coated lunch bar	382	193
2 sausages	318	286
1 individual pork pie	376	564
1 serving chip shop chips	256	670

Table 6.2

Many high-calorie foods are the ones that give us a lot of pleasure. We are not suggesting that you avoid high-calorie foods, but you must be careful to control the size of the portions you eat. Two sausages will provide you with about 285 kilocalories, but if you have four you will get 570 kilocalories. So the rule with high-calorie foods is to have smaller portion sizes. Whereas with low-calorie foods you can eat as much as you like.

It is wrong to think that only certain foods are fattening. It is commonly alleged that processed foods are more calorific. But an excess energy intake from any type of food will lead to weight-gain. There is no evidence to show that people who gain weight easily eat more sugar even though it does make many fatty foods – such as doughnuts, cakes, pastries and biscuits – taste nice. Fatty foods are more likely to make you fat because they are very high in calories and it is much easier to eat too much of them. Remember that the addition of even small amounts of fat to food can double or even treble the calorie intake. So you must be particularly careful about adding fat to food. You also need to be aware that many snack foods (for example, a packet of peanuts or a bar of chocolate) contain as many calories as a light meal.

Positive Attitudes

Some of us may need to establish better, more positive eating habits. Here are some questions to help you assess what your current attitudes to food and lifestyle are:

Q1 Meal patterns

A Do you eat one main meal and two smaller meals a day?

Usually [ ]   Occasionally [ ]   Never [ ]

B Do you eat at regular times?

Usually [ ]   Occasionally [ ]   Never [ ]

C Do you plan what you are going to eat?

Usually [ ]   Occasionally [ ]   Never [ ]

If you answered *Usually* most times, that's a good start. A regular meal pattern is essential for controlling your weight. If you answered *Occasionally* or *Never* most times, then you need to change your habits. It's better to eat your food in several small meals rather than one big one. If you don't plan what you are going to eat, it is too easy to fill up on high-calorie snacks. It also takes a lot of pleasure out of eating. Remember to stick to a regular meal pattern and you'll find the scales steady themselves.

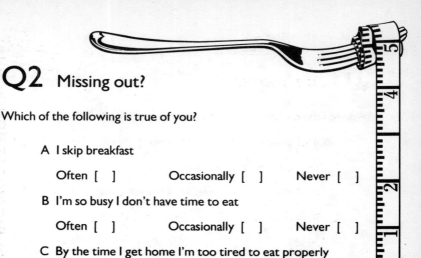

Q2 Missing out?

Which of the following is true of you?

A I skip breakfast

Often [   ] Occasionally [   ] Never [   ]

B I'm so busy I don't have time to eat

Often [   ] Occasionally [   ] Never [   ]

C By the time I get home I'm too tired to eat properly

Often [   ] Occasionally [   ] Never [   ]

If you answered *Often* or *Occasionally* to these questions, you need to establish a more stable pattern of eating. If you skip meals, you are more likely to fill up on snack foods which tend to be very high in calories. If you're at work or life is very hectic, you may find you don't have time to eat properly. If that's the case, a little forward planning is required. For example, lay out your breakfast before you go to bed and prepare a sandwich and a snack for lunch. Plan what you are going to eat for the week ahead, and choose meals that are quick to prepare but not high in fat.

Q3 The Grazer

Which of the following is true of you?   YES   NO

A I quite often stop for a snack when
   I am out shopping   [ ]   [ ]

B I usually buy some sweets or a snack to eat
   on the way to, or coming home from,
   work   [ ]   [ ]

C I often buy some food from a stall when I
   go out for a walk   [ ]   [ ]

D I usually buy something to eat in the
   car on the way home when I do the
   'big shop'   [ ]   [ ]

E I usually buy some sweets or popcorn
   when I go to the cinema   [ ]   [ ]

F I often buy sweets or snacks from
   vending machines   [ ]   [ ]

If you answered *Yes* to several of these questions it looks as if you are a grazer. Snacks and fast food can be very tempting and it can almost become a ritual if it is something you do every day, even when you are not hungry. It's interesting that many people think that food eaten standing up or outside the home doesn't count. You must learn to get out of the habit of grazing. The odd snack is all right but if you are not careful you could be consuming an additional 800 calories a day. For

154

example, a Danish pastry on the way into work, a bar of chocolate and a packet of nuts, add up to about 800 calories. At that rate you could put on a kilogram of fat in twelve days! You may be able to get away with this sort of a behaviour as a physically active and growing teenager when you need plenty of extra energy. But not as an adult!

Q4 The Home Economist

Which of the following are true of you?	YES	NO
A I always leave a clean plate	[ ]	[ ]
B I hate to see good food go to waste	[ ]	[ ]
C I find it difficult say No to free food	[ ]	[ ]

If you answered mainly *Yes*: If you want to keep control of your weight, then you have got to learn to know when you've had enough to eat. You must learn to leave food when you are full up. If you have to prepare food for other people, especially children, it is very easy to eat up the scraps even when you are not hungry. Phrases like 'Better belly bust than let good food go to waste' or 'Leave a clean plate' or 'Think of all the people starving in Ethiopia' come to mind. But you will help nobody by scoffing the leftovers. If you are on the plump side, whether it goes into your stomach or into the dustbin makes little difference except that if you eat the scraps you're asking for trouble. The rules of hospitality seem to mean that over-enthusiastic hosts press huge helpings on their guests which must then be completely consumed for fear of giving offence. This is very old-fashioned. Just say it was very nice but you're full up. And don't practise a double standard: if you're the host, don't press everybody to polish everything off, either.

Q5 Are you a Lotus Eater?

Are any of the following true of you?	YES	NO
A I often have second helpings	[ ]	[ ]
B When I have an ice-cream I usually have a big one or a double cone	[ ]	[ ]
C I like good-size portions (not like that measly *nouvelle cuisine*)	[ ]	[ ]

If you answered mainly *Yes*: You may eat too much, particularly for the pleasure of second helpings, when you're not even hungry. You need to learn to cut down on portion sizes and not to expect second helpings. Most of all, you need to listen to what your body is telling you. Eat when you are genuinely hungry. Stop eating when you are no longer hungry. Have you stopped and actually thought about this? Try it.

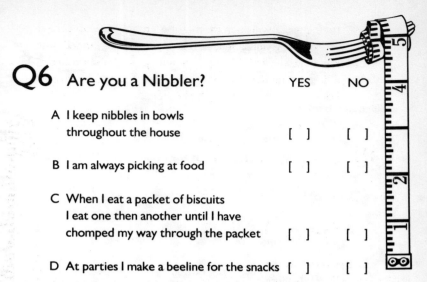

Q6 Are you a Nibbler?

		YES	NO
A	I keep nibbles in bowls throughout the house	[ ]	[ ]
B	I am always picking at food	[ ]	[ ]
C	When I eat a packet of biscuits I eat one then another until I have chomped my way through the packet	[ ]	[ ]
D	At parties I make a beeline for the snacks	[ ]	[ ]

If you answered mainly *Yes*: It sounds like you are a compulsive nibbler. Avoid nibbling at food when you are not hungry. Try to avoid situations where you will be tempted to nibble: keep away from bowls of nuts and crisps. Resist the temptation to bulk-buy snack foods like large multipacks of crisps or chocolate bars. They just encourage you to eat more. If you can't resist snack foods and biscuits if they are in the house, only buy them occasionally. Instead have an ample supply of fresh fruit to munch if you feel like a snack. If you are in the habit of 'comfort eating' (eating to make yourself feel better rather than because you are hungry), perhaps you should consider why you do it. Then you can tackle the root of the problem. What is it that is making you unhappy and in need of consolation?

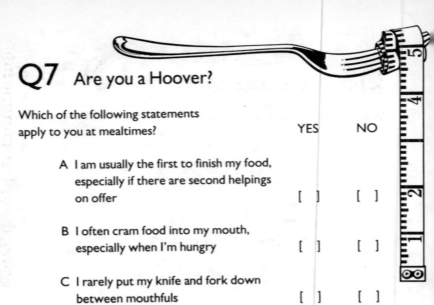

Q7 Are you a Hoover?

Which of the following statements
apply to you at mealtimes?

		YES	NO
A	I am usually the first to finish my food, especially if there are second helpings on offer	[ ]	[ ]
B	I often cram food into my mouth, especially when I'm hungry	[ ]	[ ]
C	I rarely put my knife and fork down between mouthfuls	[ ]	[ ]
D	I often eat while watching television	[ ]	[ ]

If you answered mainly *Yes*: As the comedian Tony
Hancock said, it sounds as though the food hardly touches
the sides of your throat as you eat. You might find that if
you spent a little more time eating and chewing your food,
rather than wolfing it down, you would get more pleasure
out of it. Take your time eating, make conversation.

Q8 The fat temptations

Which of the following apply to you?   YES   NO

A I can't resist those crunchy bits of
   bacon rind, or crispy roast chicken
   and pork crackling   [ ]   [ ]

B I usually spread butter/margarine
   quite thickly on bread   [ ]   [ ]

C I like my vegetables served with a
   big knob of butter   [ ]   [ ]

D I eat plenty of cheese every day   [ ]   [ ]

E I eat sausages, pies and pâté
   at least twice a week   [ ]   [ ]

F I always have at least three bags of
   crisps a week   [ ]   [ ]

G I eat plenty of salads but always with
   mayonnaise or salad cream   [ ]   [ ]

H I have a fry-up a few times a week   [ ]   [ ]

I I eat chips at least several times a week   [ ]   [ ]

If you answered *Yes* to several of these questions, you
need to watch your fat intake. Some foods like butter and
deep-fried foods are obviously fatty. But many people
don't realize that many foods like cheese, pastry and nuts

contain large amounts of hidden fat. You may eat salads regularly, but if they are swimming in mayonnaise they are very fattening. We are not saying don't eat these foods but don't eat them too often; try to use alternatives with less fat or take smaller portions.

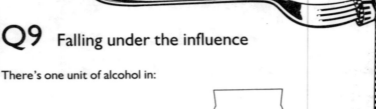

Q9 Falling under the influence

There's one unit of alcohol in:

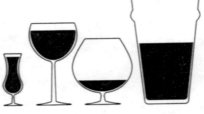

- one small glass of sherry
- one average glass of wine
- one half-pint of normal-strength beer, lager or cider
- one measure of spirits

Count up the number of units you consume a week. Experts agree that absolutely safe limits for your health are 14 units a week for women and 21 for men. But, in any case, alcoholic drinks provide plenty of calories and beer-drinking is a well known cause of obesity in men — the characteristic beer-drinker's paunch. Beer is more fattening than wine or spirits partly because it tends to be drunk in large amounts.

- 1 pint of beer provides 185 kilocalories
- 1 glass of wine provides 70 kilocalories
- 1 measure of spirits provides 50 kilocalories

But there is no need to abstain from alcohol unless of course you are pregnant, taking certain drugs or operating machinery. Indeed, moderate drinking actually helps protect from coronary heart disease.

Q10 Physically active?

		YES	NO
A	Do you spend most of the day sitting down?	[ ]	[ ]
B	Do you go by car or bus when you could walk?	[ ]	[ ]
C	Do you rarely go for a walk?	[ ]	[ ]
D	Do you take lifts rather than walk up stairs?	[ ]	[ ]
E	Do you cycle or swim regularly?	[ ]	[ ]
F	Do you play sport at least once a week?	[ ]	[ ]

If you answered *Yes* to (A), (B), (C) and (D) and *No* to (E) and (F) then you badly need to increase the level of your physical activity. Controlling weight means keeping energy intake and energy expenditure in balance. The main reason why we put on weight as we age is that we become physically less active and so are consuming more food energy than we need. We can counteract this by increasing our level of physical activity. But don't be alarmed, it only takes small changes in our everyday behaviour. Such as:

● taking the stairs instead of the lift

161

- walking or cycling rather than going by car
- swimming or aerobics classes once a week

Generally we can also take more exercise in our leisure time instead of sitting slumped in front of the television. For example, go for a long walk in the country or in the park at weekends or in the evening after work in the summer. People who remain physically active are far less likely to gain weight with age and more likely to remain fit and healthy.

Farewell to Dieting

If you have been dieting for years and put the weight back on every time you stop, then we recommend the following:

- NEVER read diet books
- NEVER buy products that claim rapid weight-loss
- NEVER take drugs or laxatives, or smoke to lose weight
- TAKE moderate exercise daily
- BUY clothes that fit comfortably
- EAT AND DRINK sensibly and enjoy your food
- EAT the same food as your family or friends — don't prepare special meals
- ACCEPT your natural shape and be comfortable with yourself

Analyse, quite honestly, whether you are generally happy or not. If there are things you are unhappy about in your life, define them and face them — don't take it out on the biscuit-tin or the bottle.

You Don't Have to Diet

In this book, we hope we have opened your eyes to the false promises of the diet industry. We have explained the complex reasons why we eat what we eat, and have shown that food, besides providing sustenance, has important meanings for us personally. Rapid weight-loss is dangerous and the pursuit of excessive slenderness is unnatural and unhealthy. There is nothing unhealthy about being plump. In fact our body build is determined in early life and there is little we can do to change it. Accepting our natural body shape is essential if we are ever to emerge from the diet trap. We explained why we put on weight and that fat is not some toxic substance accumulating in our body. We showed that fat is an essential and desirable component of human diets but to be consumed in moderation. Excessive preoccupation with food and dieting leads to eating disorders which make life miserable and can be fatal. In this last chapter, we have offered some common-sense advice about eating normally and being physically active. To achieve and maintain a comfortable healthy weight you do not need to go on a 'diet'. It happens of its own accord if you follow our advice.

So if you want to escape from the diet trap, it is up to you, and you alone. Make the right choices and take control of your life. You really don't have to diet.

7   AN A–Z OF DIETSPEAK

Allergies

Recently claims have been made that obesity may be due to food allergies, and a very restricted diet is offered as the treatment. This is scientific nonsense, and the diets prescribed are usually nutritionally unsound and encourage faddy eating. *Allergy* is the term reserved for an acute over-reaction by the immune system, usually to a protein. Allergies may be mild, as with eczema, or severe, as with anaphylactic shock. The latter can lead to collapse and death. Allergies occur for a variety of reasons but tend to run in families. Allergic individuals show responses to a variety of substances present in the environment besides food such as animal fur, dust, furnishing material, etc. Many children under the age of 3 suffer from mild food allergies but they usually grow out of them. Coeliac disease affects about 1 in 2000 children and is caused by an allergy to a protein called gluten which is found in wheat, oats, barley and rye. Allergies often lead to poor growth and weight-loss, not weight-gain, because nutrients are not properly absorbed. Other common allergies are to maize, eggs, milk, soya, shellfish, coffee, tea and chocolate. Allergies to some food additives (tartrazine, benzoates, BHT and BHA) also occur but are less common.

Allergic reactions usually appear within a few minutes but may be delayed for hours. The immediate reactions include: lip swelling, tingling of the mouth or throat, vomiting, pain or burning sensation in the stomach, difficulty breathing, runny eyes. The later reactions include diarrhoea, bloating, constipation. A proper diagnosis is essential. Don't attempt self-diagnosis or go to an 'allergy clinic' without seeing your own doctor. It is fashionable to have an allergy or for one's children to have one. The truth is that genuine allergies are less common than you might be led to believe.

Anorexia Nervosa

This literally means 'lack of appetite for nervous reasons'. The problem isn't anything to do with the food itself but the fears people have about what will happen when they eat the food. This eating disorder is mainly a female problem affecting girls and younger women. But it has also been recorded in men who are over-concerned about food for health or ethical reasons – for example, vegans. The main features of anorexia nervosa in women are excessive preoccupation with body weight and shape, fear of eating, marked interest in food and cooking, abnormal menstrual cycle (periods normally stop), loss of interest in sex, and growth of facial hair. Weight-loss can be so severe that the victim looks like something out of a concentration-camp. It is interesting that many sufferers of anorexia are good cooks and it is surprisingly common among students studying nutrition and dietetics! People with anorexia nervosa need specialized help, and medical advice should be sought (see Chapter 5).

Appetite Suppressants

These products are supposed to take away hunger pangs. Some of them are really no more than sugar pills. The idea is that if you have a little bit of sugar before a meal it will blunt your appetite. It sounds a good idea, but it doesn't work in the long run. This is because most of us don't over-eat as a result of hunger pangs. We're either greedy or over-eat out of habit.

There are also drugs that suppress appetite, but the

consensus is that, on their own, they're rarely an effective means of weight reduction. Some are addictive and may cause nasty side-effects such as high blood pressure, tiredness, diarrhoea, dry mouth and drowsiness. The Government has banned the sale of certain types of appetite suppressant drug in slimming clinics because of safety fears. Recently a large trial was carried out using one of these drugs, dexfenfluramine, versus a neutral placebo with 800 overweight adults. Both groups were given dietary advice. After six months the weight-loss was actually the same in the placebo group as with those given the drug. It's true that after a year the drug-treated group didn't regain as much weight as the placebo group. But it makes you wonder whether the patients thought it was worth putting up with the unpleasant possible side-effects of tiredness, drowsiness and diarrhoea for a year just to stop gaining a little extra weight.

Artificial Sweeteners

Artificial sweeteners are a class of food additives that fall into two categories:

- Bulk sweeteners – manitol, sorbitol, xylitol, hydrogenated glucose syrup. These have about the same calorific value as sugar and are used in many processed foods.
- Intense sweeteners – acesulfame K, aspartame, cyclamate (permitted in the EC but not in Britain), saccharin, sucralose (permitted in Canada but not yet in the EC) and thaumatin. These provide virtually no calories and are used mainly in diet drinks and tabletop sweeteners. Aspartame is the most widely used of the intense sweeteners and has a taste similar to sugar and unlike saccharin does not have a bitter aftertaste.

Soft drinks sweetened with intense sweeteners such as Diet Coke and Diet Pepsi are neither harmful to teeth nor fattening. It has been claimed that artificial sweeteners may stimulate appetite but the conclusion of most experts is that they don't. If you enjoy carbonated drinks, then it is a healthier choice to choose the low-calorie diet versions for the sake of your teeth. But don't think that by drinking diet drinks this gives you licence to over-indulge in other foods. Be sensible.

Body Mass Index

The body mass index (BMI) or Quetelet index is the method most often used to classify obesity in adults. It is calculated by dividing the weight in kilograms by the height in metres squared. For example, a man who is 85 kilograms (13 stone 5 pounds) would divide that by his height of 1.75 metres (5 foot 8½ inches) squared.

$$\frac{85}{1.75 \times 1.75} = \text{BMI of } 27.8$$

See pp.96–8 for more details

Bulimia Nervosa

Bulimia is binge-eating or stuffing yourself with food. It can occur in both fat and underweight people. It is more common in women than in men and is strongly linked to dieting. Typically there is rapid consumption of large quantities of food and drink consisting mainly of 'forbidden foods' such as biscuits, cakes, chocolate, nuts and crisps. It is then followed by a period of remorse. The individual then induces vomiting by putting a couple of fingers down their throat. But the experienced bulimic can induce vomiting at will. The whole episode is then followed by a strong feeling of guilt. See Chapter 5.

Bulking Agents

This is where the con-men have had a real field-day. They advertise pills or tablets which you take before meals to feel fuller. Generally they use such tiny amounts of the bulking agents such as guar gum or sugar beet fibre that you don't feel full, or they use so much it gives you wind and, worse still, could cause a blockage of the intestines. As a result of campaigns the Government recommended that products containing more than 15 per cent guar gum shouldn't be on sale. Some manufacturers tried to disguise the fact that they were selling guar by putting the Latin name for it (*Cyamopsis tetraglobula*) on the ingredient list. Other crafty pill-pushers have moved on to different types of gum. There is no evidence that they work; and, remember, they might gum you up.

Cellulite

This is the term used to describe the dimply fat on the tops of the legs of women. There is nothing special about cellulite – it's just a French word for fat (see page 115).

Combining Diets

One of the more recent fads is the idea that you only eat certain types of food in the same meal in order to prevent your body laying down fat. For example, it's said you shouldn't eat protein like meat with carbohydrates like bread. If you follow these rules, you're supposed to lose weight. It may sound convincing but in practice it's gobble-degook. What they don't tell you is that what they call 'carbohydrate' foods (such as bread) are also very important sources of protein in the diet. But their bizarre rules make it so difficult to eat normal meals you're bound to eat less! In reality, there are no magical combinations of foods that will make you lose weight. You can't trick your body that easily. You just have to eat fewer calories. Combining diets that offer a low-calorie regime do, indeed, help you lose weight – not because they attempt to keep foods separate but because they reduce your intake of food energy. The rest is just quackery.

Compulsive Eating

This is the term used to describe a form of addiction to eating large amounts of food even when the individual is not hungry, just for the pleasure of eating. Rather like alcoholics cannot resist drink, compulsive eaters cannot resist bingeing.

Creams

Creams have been sold with the claim that they will dissolve cellulite. One was even called 'Fadeaway', and it was alleged that all you needed to do was to rub the cream in and the fat would disappear – literally, vanishing cream. They simply do not work.

Dieting

Diet refers to the food eaten by a person or a regular pattern of eating. The word has been hijacked to mean a restricted food intake. Other basic points are:

- You will lose weight on any diet that decreases your energy intake.
- All weight-reducing diets are low in fat and alcohol.
- Crash diets claiming massive weight-loss should be avoided at all costs because they encourage faddy eating and a cycle of starvation and bingeing.

- A good diet will provide all the other nutrients you require besides calories.

The key to health is to maintain a balanced diet and a stable weight. Dieting is the problem, *not* the solution.

Diet Foods

There are thousands of products on the shelves now label-led 'low-calorie', 'reduced', 'no added sugar', or 'diet'. Legally the term 'diet' has no defined meaning. You don't have to eat special foods when you are trying to lose weight. Eating diet food on top of your ordinary diet isn't going to make you lose weight. For example, eating diet ice-cream isn't going to help you lose weight if you normally don't eat ice-cream. But diet foods can be helpful if you need to lose weight for health reasons, substituting a lower-calorie alter-native for a regular high-calorie food: for example, if you use a very low-fat spread in place of butter or margarine. Other low-calorie alternatives worth using are:

- skimmed milk in place of full cream milk
- low-fat yoghurt in place of cream
- diet soft drinks in place of sugar-sweetened drinks
- low-calorie salad dressings in place of mayonnaise or salad cream

Diuretics

Diuretics are compounds that make your body lose water and therefore (temporarily) weight. There are many herbal concoctions that have this effect and there are some drugs as well.

Some quack practitioners prescribe diuretic drugs for the treatment of obesity. This is to fool their patients into thinking that they are losing weight. Such diuretics are of no value for losing fat and may be hazardous. They can lead to the loss of essential minerals such as potassium from the body. They can also increase blood-fat levels and cause impaired blood-glucose control in people with diabetes. Many fat people are mildly diabetic, and these diuretics can make their diabetes worse.

Drugs

Various drugs are being developed that stimulate the metabolic rate (the speed at which our bodies use up nutrients to provide us with energy). Nicotine, which is present in cigarettes, increases the metabolic rate. This is why smokers tend to be lighter in weight than non-smokers and why they put on 2–3 kilograms (4.4–6.6 pounds) when they give up smoking. Other drugs known to increase metabolic rate are ephidrine and bromocryptine. All these drugs have unpleasant side-effects such as nausea and high blood pressure, and smoking causes cancer and heart disease. The drugs industry is trying to develop drugs that speed up metabolic rate but don't have the side-effects. So far they haven't been successful. At the moment several drugs are undergoing clinical trials. Even if the trials are successful, the drugs are unlikely to be available for use on patients for some years and then only for the treatment of patients with severe obesity under strict medical supervision.

Exercise

Many people are under the illusion that taking more regular exercise will make you lose lots of weight. While there are many good reasons for taking regular exercise, it only makes a small contribution to weight-loss. However, regular physical activity does help prevent you getting fat.

Fad Diets

These are diets that tell you to eat only one food – like grapefruit or bananas. If you are confined to eating any one food, then you soon get bored of it and thus limits the amount you eat. So people do lose weight over a short period on such diets. But they have no special properties.

Fasting

Starving yourself to lose weight is a very bad idea and can be quite dangerous. If you are unlucky, it can trigger an attack of gout which can be extremely painful. Some people claim they feel 'high' when they are fasting. This is because the brain switches over from using glucose as a fuel to substances called ketone bodies which are derived from the breakdown of fat. Prolonged fasting can also lead to vitamin deficiencies and can cause heart failure. Death normally results after about fifty days of fasting if water is still consumed.

Fat

Fat is the body's store of food energy – it is nature's battery. Each gram of fat yields 9 kilocalories of energy per gram. Excess food energy, whether it be from fat, carbohydrate, protein or alcohol, is stored in the body as fat. Fat also helps cushion and insulate delicate organs and is a vital structural constituent of all body organs. Fat is an essential part of human diets as it provides energy and essential fatty acids, as well as supplying and enabling the absorption of fat-soluble vitamins. Fat also makes food more palatable because it carries flavours and has a characteristic mouthfeel (see Chapter 2 and Chapter 4). Because fat is such a rich source of calories, diets high in fat are fattening. Most experts agree we should eat less fat, favouring the consumption of oils (as found in oil-rich fish, nuts, cereals, pulses and vegetable oils), rather than hard fats such as meat fat, butter, margarine and solid vegetable fats.

Fibre

A few years ago high-fibre diets were all the rage. It was claimed that if you ate a lot of fibre it would fill you up so that you wouldn't feel hungry. In the short term a bulky diet may make you feel fuller, but unfortunately most people rapidly adapt as their stomachs stretch. It is not as though wild animals that eat bulky diets have small stomachs – just think of gorillas. If you want a belly that sticks out like a gorilla, that's fine, but don't say we didn't warn you! One study compared the influence of a high intake of fibre supplements compared with placebo pills and showed a very small effect on weight-loss averaging about 40 grams (1⅓ ounces) a week. That is, it would take you six months to lose a kilogram of body weight. We should all eat a reasonable amount of fibre every day anyway. But it's decreasing our calorie intake, not mainlining on fibre, that enables us to lose weight effectively.

Many starchy foods such as bread, potatoes and beans are good sources of fibre and should be included in weight-reducing diets. But care should be taken not to eat too much of them as in excess they are fattening.

Gadgets

A variety of gadgets are on sale, such as sauna pants, massage machines and electric pads to make your muscles contract. They promise to trim your stomach, pummel your thighs or scrub up the flab. But many of these machines are a racket. You don't need a machine to take exercise, and there is certainly no reason why you should electrocute yourself!

Grapefruit

Grapefruit has no particular weight-reducing properties but it is low in calories, so you can eat as much as you like without getting fat. Grapefruit pith is a rich source of pectin, a form of dietary fibre. This led to people selling grapefruit pills claiming that they would burn off the fat. They don't work.

'Green' Diets

One of the more recent rackets has been to cash in on public awareness of environmental issues to sell 'Green' or vegetarian diets and 'Green' diet books. Excluding meat and fish from the diet does not lead to any direct weight-loss.

Guar Gum

A gum extract from the locust bean. It is used as a food additive to thicken foods. It is a form of dietary fibre and increases the feeling of satiety (see Bulking Agents). Pills containing guar gum have been sold to promote weight-loss but they are of no value.

Hormones

Hormones are substances naturally produced in the body that send messages from one organ to another. Hormones control where we deposit fat and how fast we burn it up. The female sex hormone oestrogen causes fat to be deposited around the hips and thighs. The hormone insulin stimulates the deposition of fat around the belly and shoulders. Insulin is produced in response to a meal containing starch or sugar.

Once fat is deposited it doesn't stay there for ever, it is continuously being recycled. The stress hormones adrenalin and noradrenalin control the breakdown of fat so that the body is supplied with a source of energy when it needs it. The fat stores beneath the shoulderblades, around the neck and in the belly are recycled more frequently and are more sensitive to the stress hormones than the fat stores on the hips and thighs. Consequently when the body draws on its fat reserves, those stored inside the belly, around the face, neck and shoulders are used up faster than those stored around the hips and thighs. That is, body fat is lost from the top first and the bottom last.

The thyroid hormone controls the rate at which the body uses up energy just to tick over. If too much thyroid hormone is produced, the body uses much more energy than normal. However, taking extra thyroid hormone isn't a good way to lose weight because it is accompanied by some nasty side-effects such as a very fast heartbeat and palpitations as well as mental problems.

Hypoglycaemia

This term is used to describe a low level of glucose in blood. The normal level of glucose in blood is maintained by the interaction of the hormones insulin and glucagon. If the level of blood sugar falls below this level it causes a 'cold sweat' and irritability. If it falls to very low levels, it leads to coma and death. For some people mild hypoglycaemia can occur as a rebound effect after a meal high in carbohydrates. It can also occur after bouts of drinking. Relief from mild hypoglycaemia can usually be obtained by consuming a small amount of starchy food or sugar.

Kelp Tablets

Some people claim that kelp tablets will help you lose weight because they contain iodine, which is used to make thyroid hormone. Kelp tablets have never been shown to have this effect. What's more, they may even be hazardous because too much iodine can actually damage your thyroid gland.

Laxatives

These are substances that make you empty your bowels – they cause the sort of cramps you get when you're suffering from diarrhoea. They work by irritating the lining of the gut. Some people, often those with eating disorders, take laxatives because they think it will help them lose weight. Laxatives and purgatives can cause malabsorption of nutrients leading to weight-loss and nutritional deficiencies. Some powerful laxatives like croton oil and phenolpthalein have been linked with cancer and are now banned. It is a very dangerous way to lose weight.

Lecithin

There is nothing like a scientific word to puzzle people. Lecithin is normally derived from soya beans. It is sometimes sold as a slimming aid but it is also used as a food additive (as an emulsifier to make margarine). It has been claimed that it helps mobilize fat around the body. The truth is that it has no slimming properties at all, and it is just as fattening as vegetable oil.

Liposuction

This is a surgical technique to remove fat from beneath the

skin by aspiration through a needle. It is used in cosmetic surgery. It is not an effective means of treating obesity, and if not carried out properly can lead to permanent disfiguration (*see also* Surgery).

Meal Replacements

These are usually milkshakes or snack bars that you are supposed to eat in place of real food. Currently there are no laws controlling their nutritional quality, and many are high in fat and sugar and don't provide all the nutrients required. People do lose weight if they consume them alone, but they don't change food habits and they may lead to excessive weight-loss which may do more harm than good.

Metabolism Burners or Boosters

Metabolism is the term used to describe the way in which the body uses up energy. There is a basic rate at which our body ticks over, just keeping the heart and lungs going. Some diets claim they can speed up this basic rate, rather like putting your foot on the throttle, so you burn up calories faster. Unfortunately it's not true. They don't work.

Obesity

This is the term used to describe excessive accumulation of fat inside the body. It is normally measured in terms of weight for height or body mass index. Women are naturally fatter than men. The definitions of obesity are somewhat arbitrary, and depend upon age, height and gender.

Ornithine/Arginine Combinations

There is a variety of pills being marketed at the moment that contain mixtures of amino acids. These are the basic components of proteins. One favourite combination is a mixture of ornithine and arginine. At one stage it was sold in combination with tryptophan, and the suppliers claimed that you would lose weight while you slept. These ornithine/arginine pills just don't work. We've tested them.

Spot-Reducing Fat

Some diets claim you can spot-reduce fat from your hips and thighs. This is a myth. It is not possible to manipulate the diet or to use exercise to cause fat to be lost from specific parts of the body. Some of the diets consist of avoiding fat completely. In the short term this does no harm. But a certain amount of fat is needed to enable the absorption of fat-soluble vitamins and carotene, which play a vital role in keeping us healthy.

Sprays

One of the more recent examples of the enterprise culture has been the sale of sprays that are supposed to take your appetite away. The sprays usually consist of a mixture of vitamins, amino acids and grapefruit extract. You're supposed to squirt it in your mouth when you are hungry, and the idea is that it takes your appetite away. Unfortunately, there is not a shred of evidence to show that they work. They will probably just take your breath away when you see how much they cost.

Stress

Stress can increase the rate at which you use up energy (metabolic rate) as it speeds up the heart rate. Stress can also lead to disturbed sleep as we use up less energy when we are asleep. Exposure to cold is another unpleasant way of increasing the metabolic rate at which you use up energy. Cigarette-smoking is a form of self-induced stress and it increases the metabolic rate, but it also gives you cancer and heart disease. One study looked to see if the stress induced by films affected metabolic rate. It found that metabolic rate was increased most when people watched sexy or blue films rather than horror or ordinary films!

Surgery

This is one way of losing weight we don't recommend. Some doctors offer a service called liposuction where they suck out the excess fat from under the skin. This treatment has a number of rather unpleasant side-effects and is limited in its effectiveness because you can't safely suck out fat from inside the belly without damaging some internal organs. Surgeons have even carried out operations to stop people eating as much by making their stomach smaller or to prevent them digesting the food properly by removing sections of their small intestine. Some compulsive eaters have to have their jaws wired together to stop them eating. However, many still cheat by liquidizing the food and sucking it through a straw.

Tea

There has been a variety of teas foisted on the public that have claimed to cause some weight-loss. The most famous of these was Bai-Lin, which in fact was just ordinary tea. Tea contains no calories, so if you are just drinking tea and nothing else you will lose weight. But there is nothing special in tea that makes you lose fat.

Vegetarian Diets

There has been a phenomenal increase in the number of people who claim to be vegetarians in the past four years. Vegetarian diets can be just as healthy as those of meat-eaters but the more we restrict our diet the more careful we have to be to include all the nutrients we need. *It is therefore very important that teenagers, who are also highly likely to diet, do not misuse vegetarianism merely as a way of restricting their food intake.*

It is not difficult to select a well-balanced vegetarian diet. But it is not quite as easy as one containing meat, and vegetarian meals often take more time to prepare. Cutting out certain foods doesn't necessarily make a diet healthier. Remember, the quality of any diet depends on what foods are included, not on those left out. Usually the first stage in becoming a vegetarian is to give up eating red meat and this is followed by cutting out poultry and fish. But there are degrees of vegetarianism. Generally the term *vegetarian* is used to describe those who include eggs and dairy products in their diet. *Vegans*, or strict vegetarians, eat no foods of animal origin whatsoever. *Fruitarians* are the most extreme, eating only raw fruit, nuts and berries. Vegetarian and vegan diets can be quite healthy providing they are properly planned. Fruitarian diets can lead to severe nutritional deficiencies and are best avoided.

If you are not eating a very good diet anyway and you give up meat and don't compensate for it by using healthy vegetarian alternatives, then you could have problems. For example, a diet comprising sweets, crisps, chips, biscuits and beer isn't a good vegetarian diet. Nutritional deficiencies are much more likely to occur in children than in adults because they are growing.

The two main pitfalls to watch out for when becoming a vegetarian are:

- depending too heavily on fatty and sweet refined foods, like biscuits, which are poor sources of other nutrients
- not getting enough vitamin B_{12} and iron

Choosing a well-balanced vegetarian diet is much easier if it is based round good staple foods such as wholemeal bread, pasta, potatoes or rice. Using wholemeal cereals also ensures a high intake of fibre, iron and B-complex vitamins. These nutrients are then complemented by those provided in milk products, eggs, fruit and vegetables to add all the other nutrients required.

The last word on vegetarianism is that it can and should be perfectly healthy. But only if those practising it do so carefully so as to ensure they get all the nutrients they need. It should never be an excuse for faddy eating.

Very Low Calorie Diets

These are a form of meal replacement that usually provide up to 600 calories per day in the form of milkshakes or snack bars. They lead to rapid weight-loss, and experts agree they should not be used except under strict medical supervision in view of the hazards associated with their use (see Chapter 1 and Chapter 4).

Vitamin and Mineral Supplements

There is no evidence that supplements help you lose weight. If you eat a good diet there should be no need to take supplements. But if you do want to take a supplement at a reasonable dose it won't do you any harm. If you are a vegan, housebound or anaemic you may need to take supplements. But remember: because small amounts of vitamins and minerals are good for you, larger amounts aren't necessarily better, and can even be poisonous. If you take supplements, choose those that provide an amount equivalent to the recommended daily amounts of all the nutrients. Treat them like medicines and do *not* exceed the stated doses.

Yo-Yo Diets

These are diets that encourage a cycle of fasting and binge-ing. You starve yourself one week and pig out the next week. Drastic changes in diet are bad news. If you want to lose weight, then you should aim to do it gently and change those habits that led to you being overweight in the first place.

INDEX

Page numbers in bold represent items in the A–Z of Dietspeak.

189